T0312181

Psychological Insights for Understanding COVID-19 and Media and Technology

In the *Psychological Insights for Understanding COVID*-19 series, international experts introduce important themes in psychological science that engage with people's unprecedented experience of the pandemic, drawing together chapters as they originally appeared before COVID-19 descended on the world.

This book explores how COVID-19 has impacted our relationship with media and technology, and chapters examine a range of topics including fake news, social media, conspiracy theories, belonging, online emotional lives and relationship formation and identity. It shows the benefits media and technology can have in relation to coping with crises and navigating challenging situations, whilst also examining the potential pitfalls that emerge due to our increasing reliance on them. In a world where the cyberpsychological space is constantly developing, this volume exposes the complexities surrounding the interaction of human psychology with media and technology, and reflects on what this might look like in the future.

Featuring theory and research on key topics germane to the global pandemic, the *Psychological Insights for Understanding COVID-19* series offers thought-provoking reading for professionals, students, academics and policy makers concerned with the psychological consequences of COVID-19 for individuals, families and society.

Ciarán Mc Mahon, Ph.D., is a director of the Institute of Cyber Security, author of *The Psychology of Social Media,* and co-author of *Cyber Security ABCs: Delivering Awareness, Behaviours and Culture Change.*

Psychological Insights for Understanding COVID-19

The *Psychological Insights for Understanding COVID-19* series aims to highlight important themes in psychological science that engage with people's unprecedented experience of the COVID-19 pandemic. These short, accessible volumes draw together chapters as they originally appeared before COVID-19 descended on the world but demonstrate how researchers and professionals in psychological science had developed theory and research on key topics germane to the global pandemic. Each volume includes a specially commissioned, expert introduction that contextualises the chapters in relation to the crisis, reflects on the relevance of psychological research during this significant global event, and proposes future research and vital interventions that elucidate understanding and coping with COVID-19. With individual volumes exploring society, health, family, work and media, the *Psychological Insights for Understanding COVID-19* series offers thought-provoking reading for professionals, students, academics and policy makers concerned with psychological consequences of the pandemic for individuals, families and society.

Titles in the series:

Psychological Insights for Understanding COVID-19 and Families, Parents, and Children
Edited by Marc H. Bornstein

Psychological Insights for Understanding COVID-19 and Media and Technology
Edited by Ciarán Mc Mahon

Psychological Insights for Understanding COVID-19 and Society
Edited by S. Alexander Haslam

Psychological Insights for Understanding COVID-19 and Work
Edited by Cary L. Cooper

Psychological Insights for Understanding COVID-19 and Health
Edited by Dominika Kwasnicka and Robbert Sanderman

For more information about this series, please visit: www.routledge.com/ Psychological-Insights-for-Understanding-COVID-19/book-series/COVID

Psychological Insights for Understanding COVID-19 and Media and Technology

Edited by Ciarán Mc Mahon

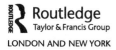
Routledge
Taylor & Francis Group

LONDON AND NEW YORK

First published 2021
by Routledge
2 Park Square, Milton Park, Abingdon, Oxon OX14 4RN

and by Routledge
52 Vanderbilt Avenue, New York, NY 10017

Routledge is an imprint of the Taylor & Francis Group, an informa business

British Library Cataloguing-in-Publication Data
A catalogue record for this book is available from the British Library

Library of Congress Cataloging-in-Publication Data
A catalog record for this book has been requested

ISBN: 978-0-367-64007-1 (hbk)
ISBN: 978-0-367-64006-4 (pbk)
ISBN: 978-1-003-12175-6 (ebk)

Typeset in Times New Roman
by Apex CoVantage, LLC

Selected chapters are taken from the following original Routledge publications

The Psychology of Fake News: Accepting, Sharing, and Correcting Misinformation
Rainer Greifeneder, Mariela Jaffe, Eryn Newman, Norbert Schwarz
ISBN: 978-0-367-27181-7 (hbk) ISBN: 978-0-367-27183-1 (pbk) ISBN: 978-0-429-29537-9 (ebk)

The Psychology of Social Media
Ciarán Mc Mahon
ISBN: 978-1-138-04774-7 (hbk) ISBN: 978-1-138-04775-4 (pbk) ISBN: 978-1-315-17061-9 (ebk)

The Psychology of Conspiracy Theories
Jan-Willem van Prooijen
ISBN: 978-1-138-69609-9 (hbk) ISBN: 978-1-138-69610-5 (pbk) ISBN: 978-1-315-52541-9 (ebk)

An Introduction to Cyberpsychology
Irene Connolly, Marion Palmer, Hannah Barton, Gráinne Kirwan
ISBN: 978-1-138-82378-5 (hbk) ISBN: 978-1-138-82379-2 (pbk) ISBN: 978-1-315-74189-5 (ebk)

The Psychology of Belonging
Kelly-Ann Allen
ISBN: 978-0-367-34753-6 (hbk) ISBN: 978-0-367-34752-9 (pbk) ISBN: 978-0-429-32768-1 (ebk)

Applications of Social Psychology: How Social Psychology Can Contribute to the Solution of Real-World Problems
Joseph P. Forgas, William D. Crano, Klaus Fiedler
ISBN: 978-0-367-41832-8 (hbk) ISBN: 978-0-367-41833-5 (pbk) ISBN: 978-0-367-81640-7 (ebk)

Wired Youth: The Online Social World of Adolescence, Second Edition
Ilan Talmud, Gustavo Mesch
ISBN: 978-0-8153-7883-9 (hbk) ISBN: 978-0-8153-7884-6 (pbk) ISBN: 978-1-351-22774-2 (ebk)

Emergent Identities: New Sexualities, Genders and Relationships in a Digital Era
Rob Cover
ISBN: 978-1-138-09858-9 (hbk) ISBN: 978-1-138-09861-9 (pbk) ISBN: 978-1-315-10434-8 (ebk)

Contents

Contributors

Kelly-Ann Allen, School of Education, Monash University, Australia, drkellyallen@gmail.com

Susannah Chandhok, Graduate Student, Department of Psychology, University of Michigan, susac@umich.edu

Rob Cover, Media and Communication Studies, University of Western Australia, Australia, rob.cover@uwa.edu.au

Olivia Hurley, Institute of Art, Design + Technology (IADT), Ireland, Olivia.Hurley@iadt.ie

Madeline Jalbert, Graduate Student, Department of Psychology, University of Southern California, Los Angeles, USA, mcjalber@usc.edu

Ethan Kross, Department of Psychology, University of Michigan, USA, ekross@umich.edu

Gustavo Mesch, Department of Sociology, University of Haifa, Israel, gustavo@soc.haifa.ac.il

Norbert Schwarz, Department of Psychology, University of Southern California, Los Angeles, USA, norberts@usc.edu

Ilan Talmud, Department of Sociology, University of Haifa, Israel talmud@soc.haifa.ac.il

Jan-Willem van Prooijen, Department of Experimental and Applied Psychology, VU Amsterdam, Netherlands, j.w.van.prooijen@vu.nl

Introduction

Ciarán Mc Mahon

I hope this finds you well

'In these extraordinary times' seems like a trite understatement, but it has become a common phrase in emails in 2020. Conventional language seems redundant given the horror of the COVID-19 pandemic. Similarly, it can feel peculiar to be still writing and reading about such abstract things as media psychology. But our way of life must somehow continue, as soon as we have completed the more fundamental task of surviving.

In a generally prescient study of the psychology of pandemics, Taylor (2019, p. 108) writes, "If the next pandemic is like some past pandemics in which children and young adults were most susceptible, then there will be many parents grieving for their lost children." Thankfully this has not come to pass, as children do not appear to be especially susceptible to this virus. But I suspect that many parents of school-goers are currently experiencing something akin to grief – grief for their offspring's childhood – friendships disrupted, habits broken, learning interrupted. A vast unexpected experiment in home-schooling and working-from-home has been dropped on a large portion of the population, and most of us do not quite know what has hit us – perhaps we should instead be talking about living at school, or homing at work. This new normal has driven a coach-and-four into lots of social concepts – from work/life balance to screen time and presumably many more besides.

In whatever future we had been imagining, a chasm of vantablack has appeared. Nothing like this has happened in living memory – we are in utterly unchartered territory. This is true in almost every human or social science direction we care to gaze, but perhaps exceptionally so when we think of the cyberpsychological space – the complicated interaction of human psychology with our various forms of media and technology. In itself, this is a new and exciting field of scholarly activity. For researchers in this area, almost everything is still 'to be decided'. There are few settled questions, and novel controversies emerge practically with each passing week.

Yet at the same time, there is no way out of this pandemic without an increasingly complicated and mediated future. Throughout society a 'data feeding frenzy' has begun – even into our beloved pubs (Walsh, 2020) as patrons record their personal details for contact tracing purposes. A boom in workplace surveillance is happening as employers roll out temperature checks and try to predict employees' risk of infection (Chyi, 2020). As more people work from home, bosses are 'panic-buying' surveillance software, snapping screenshots of their remote employees (Mosendz & Melin, 2020). Many of these workers are also parents, whose home schooling experience has been repeatedly described as 'hell' (Cassidy, 2020; Krishan, 2020; Sellgren, 2020). In an excruciating example of a deepening digital divide, the BBC (2020) reported one family attempting to home-school six children on a single phone – and they are surely not alone.

And when those of us who do have the luxury of our own personal devices do finally get a chance to relax of an evening, we may realise that our favourite content creators are also feeling the pinch. Online advertising revenues are falling due to a collapsing economy, while competition for viewers increases as everyone from TV celebrities to the average Joe films their daily experience of the pandemic (Lorenz, 2020). As hard as it is to imagine, the internet is now even more awash with content than it was before.

It feels appropriate to quote Marshall McLuhan (1967, p. 94): "These are difficult times because we are witnessing a clash of cataclysmic proportions between two great technologies. We approach the new with the psychological conditioning and sensory responses of the old." It is the natural instinct of a researcher, when encountering a new problem, to see how previous comparable problems were cracked. Unhelpfully, we seem to know little about the wider societal impact of the last global pandemic, namely the so-called Spanish Flu. Perhaps this is because it occurred during a wartime era, with strict controls on publicity and little budget for reflexive scholarship. Or maybe people wanted to forget about it? Perhaps we will want to forget about this one, but I doubt we will be able to.

Crucially, I suspect we will be studying the technological aspects of this moment for quite some time. This is because that context was already within a cultural moment of significant angst, beginning with the Snowden revelations in 2013, right through the Cambridge Analytica controversy of 2018 and several other scandals in between. Furthermore, this period's woes will now be crystallised in our 'technologies of memory' like Wikipedia (Betuel, 2020). Whether we would like to forget it or not, all aspects of the COVID-19 pandemic will be recorded digitally, and how those records are managed and updated will affect in turn how we psychologically remember this pandemic.

However, this unrest is much more in evidence with regard to profit-generating tech services than non-profits like Wikipedia. It is something of an understatement to say that over the last five to ten years, the global community has been unnerved by the increasing power of the major tech corporations – in spite of their extraordinary abilities to create technologies that so many of us seem to love using every day. Consequently, this pandemic moment has presented an acute challenge to the likes of Apple, Google and Microsoft.

Some commentators have opined that while a moment of redemption may have presented itself for such companies, it seems to have passed. At the beginning of the crisis, "screens were no longer an addictive distraction from real life, but the locus of real life itself" (Oremus, 2020). But that moment passed when a host of regulatory and political concerns reared their head once more. For example, a trust deficit (Fung, 2020) has emerged for Facebook, with large numbers of advertisers departing its services due to its handling of misinformation and hate speech issues. Furthermore, at the beginning of the crisis, social media users all across the world noticed something strange happening to their newsfeeds. Favourite accounts suddenly disappeared, and innocuous content was unexplainably marked as spam and removed. As Facebook, Twitter and YouTube sent human content moderators home (Matsakis & Martineau, 2020), the algorithms were left in control, and the result was not pretty.

The irony is that we are now being asked to place our trust in technology to at least partially get us out of this mess. As I mentioned in *The Psychology of Social Media* (Mc Mahon, 2019) an essential truth about social media services is that they encourage users to commodify themselves – their personal information, their emotions, their sociality – and put it online. This is a reality that most of us feel uncomfortable about on the rare occasion when we pause to examine it. But now in 2020, we are being asked to share our location and interaction history with contact tracing apps, where the personal information is gathered for the purpose of saving lives. Will this feel less unpleasant, because we're not generating private profit but attempting to help the greater good? Or will it feel more like the consolidation of this unease, a normalisation of this model of commodification and surveillance?

Despite the fact that "tech-based solutions being pursued and deployed are far from ideal and have a number of issues that suggest they may not be fit-for-purpose" (Kitchin, 2020, p. 7), such smartphone applications are being pushed out by governments all across the world in an attempt to halt the spread of the coronavirus. In that light, the failure of many advanced nations, including the United Kingdom, to build such an app without the involvement help of Google and Apple (Sabbagh & Hern, 2020) is remarkable. What does that say about state capacity to protect its citizens in the technology sphere? As one scholar has queried, even if these tech giants get everything right about the privacy aspects of these apps, is there still something fundamentally wrong (Sharon, 2020)? We are now at a point where tech corporations' involvement in modern life has moved from the useful to the essential: it is difficult to see how societies can now function without them.

Treatments

In this volume, we have put together a selection of scholarship which, while not explicitly about this crisis, is as close to that intellectual neighbourhood as one could hope to be. It is hoped that the enormity of this crisis can be better understood by reflecting on the individual's experience of it – how we try to navigate and make sense of this world with the technologies around us.

Chapter 1, titled "When (Fake) News Feels True: Intuitions of Truth and the Acceptance and Correction of Misinformation," comes from Norbert Schwarz and Madeline Jalbert (2021) and could not be a more apposite example of this. The pandemic has spawned an explosion of news coverage as scared citizens search for accurate information about this new and unknown threat. However, this crisis is spawning an equally vast explosion of untruths. Research has observed that major producers of disinformation tend to produce less content than professional media organisations, but they can attract as much as 10 times the level of online engagement with their content (Howard, 2020). In Schwarz and Jalbert's chapter we understand why this is concerning. Essentially, the conditions necessary for correcting misconceptions, such as interested recipients, with time to consider the counter-messaging and with some incentives too, contrast signficantly with the reality of public information campaigns, where social media users are continually bombarded with all kinds of conflicting information and enticements. Policy makers attempting to counteract the COVID-19 infodemic would do well to consider this chapter in detail.

Our second chapter, "Connections," comes from my own *The Psychology of Social Media* (2019). Here I discuss the benefits and drawbacks which we experience on social media from being able to connect with lots of people in a single space. For example, research has shown that users of Facebook and Snapchat benefit differently from either site. That is, knowing that some social media sites can help users develop bridging social capital, while others help more with bonding social capital, can help researchers better understand how social media users may be coping during the pandemic. For example, has physical distancing affected what users want from their social media services? Has that contributed to the increased popularity of TikTok?

I also discuss Dunbar's numbers within social media studies, and in particular the lesser-known ones, namely the sympathy group and the support clique. This treatment may be useful with regard to, for example, the mutual aid groups which have sprung up in many locations (Butler, 2020). Another concept discussed here is that of FOMO – or the fear of missing out. How has this phenomenon evolved during the pandemic? Media outlets are reporting conflicting experiences, with some saying that the lockdown has "cured their FOMO" (Burleigh, 2020) while others admit that while they feel bad about it, they are still experiencing fear of missing out (Tait, 2020).

In Chapter 3, we come to "When Do People Believe Conspiracy Theories?" by Jan-Willem van Prooijen (2018). He quickly dismisses the idea that our modern internet is somehow more conducive to belief in conspiracies. On the contrary, van Prooijen shows that it is in fact societal crisis situations, not any particular aspect of the media landscape, which give rise to this kind of thinking – an apt illustration in these times.

Startlingly, this chapter contains a very prescient section, asking the reader to imagine what would happen if a head of government fell ill or died with a flu virus. Would the public believe that their illness was indeed caused by a medical condition, or would they prefer a conspiracy theory of some kind? In fact, as we have seen, when Prime Minister Johnson fell ill with COVID-19 (and thankfully recovered unlike in van Prooijen's example), conspiracy theories immediately flourished. Not only did a Downing Street spokesperson have to deny disinformation claims that he was going to be put on a ventilator (McGuinness, 2020), but reports also circulated that not only was Johnson not really sick, but that staff at the hospital where he was being treated had to sign the Official Secrets Act to that effect (Milne, 2020). All of which is false, and all of which only further serves to illustrate van Prooijen's point in this chapter: that conspiracy theories are basically natural reactions to social situations of fear and uncertainty. I suspect that this is something that many of us know but have not paused to admit: for the last few months, we have been living in dread, with none of the normal confidence about the future. Consequently, it is inevitable that conspiracy theories would spring up at this time. As van Prooijen explains: "Sense making thus is essential in the psychology of conspiracy theories."

The fourth chapter in this volume is Olivia Hurley's "The Dynamics of Groups Online" (2016). In the 'before times', this would have been an interesting chapter. Today, as vast amounts of our socialising have been forced online, it becomes an essential read. I note, for example, Hurley's sketching of the most common reasons for joining online groups, including 'alleviating loneliness' – "whether that is temporary, such as moving to a new city, or chronic, such as being housebound for long periods of time". When researchers come to examine online sociality during the lockdown, will they find that we have joined lots more online groups than usual? Similarly, the pandemic has brought a variety of new online organising tools for communities (Brechter, 2020), so researchers and practitioners will be eager to apply concepts from this chapter, such as online group cohesion, social loafing and groupthink to their contexts. Has the lockdown exacerbated – or intensified? – these phenomena?

The meme 'Congratulations, you survived a meeting that could have been an email' leads off our fifth chapter, Kelly-Ann Allen's "Belonging in an Age of Technology" (2021). This came to life for many people working remotely over the last few months as lots of meetings did in fact become emails. The point Allen makes is not a trivial one though – in the 21st century we have lots of ways of connecting with each other, but is this technology helping or hindering our sense of belonging?

In exploring how communication technology has become the 'bricks and mortar of our daily existence', Allen gives us a useful treatment of the concept of 'screen time', which has surely taken a battering over the last few months. As many of us have worked and schooled from home recently, our patterns of technology use have surely drastically altered, but also our sense of belonging. A relatively new practice which has exploded during the lockdown period in many countries is the phenomenon of the watchparty (Wallenstein, 2020) – where people in separate locations can chat together online while watching the same TV show or movie. Can we be alone together, via Netflix? As Allen carefully explains, this depends not only how we define belonging, but also how we manage the process of technological change.

Next we come to Ethan Kross and Susannah Chandhok's chapter, "How Do Online Social Networks Influence People's Emotional Lives?" (2020). This piece confronts perhaps the most essential debate in media psychology. How come, on the one hand, many studies reveal negative associations between emotional well-being and social media usage, whereas on the other, many reveal positive associations? This they term *The Puzzle* – a conceptual and methodological challenge which will likely intensify in the post-pandemic world.

Helpfully, Kross and Chandhok address questions such as 'Why do people continue to use social media if doing so consistently leads them to feel worse?' and 'Are there ways of harnessing social media to improve well-being?' We can see aspects of this during this lockdown. For many of us logging on to social media in 2020 may have been quite a deflating, if not depressing, experience, with wave after wave of terrible news. Yet at the same time, through hashtags and memes such as #inthistogether, 'flattening the curve' and 'stay home save lives', perhaps we found ways to influence our own emotions on social media by attempting to help each other.

In our seventh chapter, we move to online relationship formation in young people, by Ilan Talmud and Gustavo Mesch (2020). This piece contains pressing analysis for those working with teens and young people. Their focus here is on the similarities, differences and overlap between online and offline social relationships in adolescents.

A recent viewpoint in *The Lancet* makes the point that the physical distancing measures put in place to prevent the spread of COVID-19 will have removed face-to-face contact from social connection, thereby disrupting the peer-to-peer interaction at the heart of adolescent well-being (Orben, Tomova, & Blakemore, 2020). The authors suggest that use of digital technologies may mitigate this disruption and that further research is urgently necessary.

In their chapter, Talmud and Mesch give us some clues as to how this mitigation may occur and what researchers should look out for. They note that while research shows that online friendships are regularly perceived to be lower in quality than offline friendships, the quality of online friendships improves significantly more so than do offline relationships. Perhaps social distancing may in fact produce stronger online friendships for teens? Crucially however, Talmud and Mesch argue that the very concept of 'online relationship' itself requires clarification, which is something researchers must address in the post-pandemic context.

During the last few months, along with everything else we have gone through, many of us will have gained new aspects to our psychological identities. Some of us will have become 'cocooners', 'shielders' or 'compromised' – and preliminary research warns of potential divides between 'distancers' and 'non-distancers' (Prosser, Judge, Bolderdijk, Blackwood, & Kurz, 2020). Strikingly, in the United States the very act of wearing a mask has become endowed with political symbolism (Hess, 2020).

As such, it is very useful to conclude this volume with "Identity Citizenship" by Rob Cover (2019). While this chapter is largely concerned with sexual and gender identities, we can also see how this work is acutely relevant in the post-pandemic context. In particular, Cover begins by showing while new ways of thinking about sexuality and gender first appear online, it is not really useful to think of digital media as causing these new ideas to emerge. Rather, he argues we should consider the cultural conditions which give rise to such ideas. Of the cultural factors he incorporates into this analysis, the 'cult of authenticity' and the 'role of populism' strike me as of being highly relevant in how we come to understand ourselves in the new normal.

To conclude, all has changed, changed utterly, a terrible beauty has once again been born. At time of writing (July 2020) it is far from clear what new future will emerge from this crisis, nor how much of the past will survive. I hope in this Introduction I have adequately shown, however, that our new lives will most certainly be mediated by the complicated interaction of human psychology and information technology – moreover, that the chapters which follow will be useful in understanding that context. It is understanding the issues which are covered in subsequent pages – from fake news and conspiracy theories, to our identities and emotions, our sense of belonging and online groups, connections and relationships – which will be crucial to how we survive within an increasingly mediated post-COVID-19 world.

References

Allen, K.-A. (2021). *The psychology of belonging*. London: Routledge.

BBC News. (2020, May 19). Homeschooling six children with just one phone. *BBC News*. Retrieved from https://www.bbc.com/news/av/education-52717519/coronavirus-homeschooling-six-children-with-just-one-phone

Betuel, E. (2020, June 23). How the internet will change our coronavirus memories. *Inverse*. Retrieved from https://www.inverse.com/mind-body/COVID19-memory-history

Brechter, H. A. (2020, April 8). In coronavirus pandemic, groups use online tools to fight isolation. *USA Today*. Retrieved from https://eu.usatoday.com/story/opinion/2020/04/07/coronavirus-pandemic-groups-use-online-tools-fight-isolation-column/5090452002/

Burleigh, N. (2020, May 3). Fomo haunted me for years – but the coronavirus pandemic cured me. *The Guardian*. Retrieved from https://www.theguardian.com/commentis-free/2020/may/03/coronavirus-pandemic-fomo-vanity

Butler, P. (2020, March 16). COVID-19 Mutual Aid: how to help vulnerable people near you. *The Guardian*. Retrieved from https://www.theguardian.com/world/2020/mar/16/COVID-19-mutual-aid-how-to-help-the-vulnerable-near-you

Cassidy, A. (2020, April 28). Homeschooling hell: "I'm under so much pressure and it's from the mums" WhatsApp groups'. *Image*. Retrieved from https://www.image.ie/life/homeschooling-hell-im-much-pressure-mums-whatsapp-groups-187142

Chyi, N. (2020, May 12). The workplace-surveillance technology boom. *Slate*. Retrieved from https://slate.com/technology/2020/05/workplace-surveillance-apps-coronavirus.html

Cover, R. (2019). *Emergent identities*. London: Routledge.

Fung, B. (2020). Facebook exec admits there is a "trust deficit" as advertiser boycott accelerates. *CNN Business*. Retrieved from https://edition.cnn.com/2020/06/24/tech/facebook-trust-deficit/index.html

Hess, A. (2020, June 2). The Medical Mask Becomes a Protest Symbol. *The New York Times*. Retrieved from https://www.nytimes.com/2020/06/02/arts/virus-mask-trump.html

Howard, P. N. (2020). Bending the Curve of Fake Pandemic News. *Project Syndicate*. Retrieved from https://www.project-syndicate.org/commentary/much-COVID19-disinformation-traceable-to-authoritarian-regimes-by-philip-n-howard-2020–06

Hurley, O. (2016). The dynamics of groups online. In I. Connolly, M. Palmer, H. Barton, & G. Kirwan (Eds.), *An Introduction to Cyberpsychology* (pp. 98–110). Oxford: Routledge. https://doi.org/10.4324/9781315741895-18

Kitchin, R. (2020). Civil liberties or public health, or civil liberties and public health? Using surveillance technologies to tackle the spread of COVID-19. *Space and Polity*, *0*(0), 1–20. https://doi.org/10.1080/13562576.2020.1770587

Krishan, P. (2020, May 26). The reality of homeschooling has been an experience from hell - and it's affected my son too. *INews*. Retrieved from https://inews.co.uk/opinion/the-reality-of-homeschooling-has-been-an-experience-from-hell-and-its-affecting-my-son-too-431220

Kross, E., & Chandhok, S. (2020). *Applications of social psychology*. London: Routledge. https://doi.org/10.4324/9780367816407-13

Lorenz, T. (2020). Influencing? In This Economy? It's Only Gotten More Competitive. Retrieved June 25, 2020, from https://www.nytimes.com/2020/04/23/style/creator-coach-influencers-coronavirus.html

Matsakis, L., & Martineau, P. (2020, March 18). Coronavirus Disrupts Social Media's First Line of Defense. *Wired*. Retrieved from https://www.wired.com/story/coronavirus-social-media-automated-content-moderation/

Mc Mahon, C. (2019). *The psychology of social media*. London: Routledge. https://doi.org/10.4324/9781315170619

McGuinness, A. (2020, April 6). Coronavirus: Downing Street slams Russian "disinformation" over Boris Johnson ventilator claim. *Sky News*. Retrieved from https://news.sky.com/story/coronavirus-downing-street-slams-russian-disinformation-over-boris-johnson-ventilator-claim-11969398

McLuhan, M. (1967). *The medium is the massage*. London: Penguin.

Milne, C. (2020, April 15). False posts that suggest Boris Johnson didn't have COVID-19 are based on a blog post now labelled as satire. *Full Fact*. Retrieved from https://fullfact.org/online/false-post-boris-johnson-hospital-official-secrets/

Mosendz, P., & Melin, A. (2020). Bosses Panic-Buy Spy Software to Keep Tabs on Remote Workers. *Bloomberg*. Retrieved from https://www.bloomberg.com/news/features/2020-03-27/bosses-panic-buy-spy-software-to-keep-tabs-on-remote-workers

Orben, A., Tomova, L., & Blakemore, S. J. (2020). The effects of social deprivation on adolescent development and mental health. *The Lancet Child and Adolescent Health*, *4*(8), 634–640. https://doi.org/10.1016/S2352-4642(20)30186-3

Oremus, W. (2020). Will Tech's Monopolies Survive 2020? *OneZero*. Retrieved from https://onezero.medium.com/will-techs-monopolies-survive-2020-90a8ea05b6c3

Prosser, A. M. B., Judge, M., Bolderdijk, J. W., Blackwood, L., & Kurz, T. (2020). 'Distancers' and 'non-distancers'? The potential social psychological impact of moralizing COVID-19 mitigating practices on sustained behaviour change. *British Journal of Social Psychology*, *59*, 653–662. https://doi.org/10.1111/bjso.12399

Sabbagh, D., & Hern, A. (2020, June 18). UK abandons contact-tracing app for Apple and Google model. *The Guardian*. Retrieved from https://www.theguardian.com/world/2020/jun/18/uk-poised-to-abandon-coronavirus-app-in-favour-of-apple-and-google-models

Schwarz, N., & Jalbert, M. (2021). When (Fake) News Feels True: Intutions of Truth and the Acceptance and Correction of Misinformation. In R. Greifeneder, M. Jaffe, E. Newman, & N. Schwarz (Eds.), *The Psychology of Fake News*. London: Routledge.

Sellgren, K. (2020, July 8). Coronavirus: Home-schooling has been hell, say parents. *BBC News*. Retrieved from https://www.bbc.com/news/education-53319615

Sharon, T. (2020). When Google and Apple get privacy right, is there still something wrong? Retrieved June 25, 2020, from https://medium.com/@TamarSharon/when-google-and-apple-get-privacy-right-is-there-still-something-wrong-a7be4166c295

Tait, A. (2020, April 16). Is everyone partying on Zoom without me? *PaperMag*. Retrieved from https://www.papermag.com/quarantine-fomo-zoom-parties-2645734658.html

Talmud, I., & Mesch, G. (2020). *Wired youth: The online social world of adolescence* (2nd ed.). London: Routledge.

Taylor, S. (2019). *The psychology of pandemics*. Cambridge: Cambridge Scholars Publishing.

van Prooijen, J.-W. (2018). *The psychology of conspiracy theories*. London: Routledge.

Wallenstein, A. (2020, June 24). "Watch Party" Trend Sweeping the Video World Amid Lockdown. *Variety*. Retrieved from https://variety.com/2020/digital/news/watch-party-video-trend-coronavirus-1234643586/

Walsh, R. (2020). Details at the pub door: COVID is becoming a data feeding frenzy. Retrieved June 25, 2020, from https://www.politics.co.uk/comment-analysis/2020/06/25/details-at-the-pub-door-covid-is-becoming-a-data-feeding-fre

1

WHEN (FAKE) NEWS FEELS TRUE

Intuitions of truth and the acceptance and correction of misinformation

Norbert Schwarz and Madeline Jalbert

An analysis of 2.8 million episodes of news sharing on Twitter found that 59% of the news items were shared without having been opened (Gabielkov, Ramach-andran, Chaintreau, & Legout, 2016). Apparently, six out of ten readers found the headline compelling enough to share the piece without reading it. In this chapter, we review what makes a message "feel" true, even before we have considered its content in any detail. We first discuss the basic psychological processes involved in assessing the truth of a message and illustrate them with select experiments. Subsequently, we address the implications of these processes for information sharing on social media and the correction of misinformation.

Evaluating truth

While retweeting something without reading it may strike many readers as surprising and irresponsible, it is not distinctly different from how we communicate in everyday life. In daily conversations, we proceed on the tacit assumption that the speaker is a cooperative communicator whose contributions are relevant to the ongoing conversation, truthful, informative, and clear (Grice, 1975; Sperber & Wilson, 1986). Unless we have reason to doubt that the speaker observes these tacit rules of conversational conduct, we accept the content of the utterance without much questioning and treat it as part of the common ground of the conversation. These conversational processes contribute to many errors in human judgment (for reviews, see Schwarz, 1994, 1996). Some research even suggests that comprehension of a statement requires at least temporary acceptance of its truth (Gilbert, 1991) before it can be checked against relevant evidence.

While suspension of belief is possible (Hasson, Simmons, & Todorov, 2005; Schul, Mayo, & Burnstein, 2008), it requires implausibility of the message or distrust at the time it is received. Hence, the deck is usually stacked in favor of accepting information rather than rejecting it, provided there are no salient markers that call the speaker's cooperativeness into question. Going beyond the default of information acceptance requires motivation and cognitive resources, which we are most likely to invest when the topic is important to us and there are few competing demands and distractions. In the absence of these conditions, information is likely to be accepted – and sometimes passed on – without much scrutiny.

When people do evaluate whether information is likely to be true, they typically consider some (but rarely all) of the five criteria shown in Table 5.1 (Schwarz, 2015). Is the claim compatible with other things they know? Is it internally consistent and coherent? Does it come from a trustworthy source? Do other people agree with it? Is there much evidence to support it? Each of these criteria is sensible and does, indeed, bear on the likely truth of a message. These criteria can be assessed by considering relevant knowledge, which is a relatively slow and effortful process and may require extensive information search. The same criteria can also be assessed by relying on one's intuitive response, which is faster and less taxing. When the initial intuitive response suggests that something may be wrong, people are likely to turn to the more effortful analysis, provided time and circumstances allow for it. This makes initial intuitive assessments of truth a key gatekeeper for whether people will further engage with the message using a critical eye or just nod along in agreement. These assumptions are compatible with a long history of research in social (e.g., Petty & Cacioppo, 1986) and cognitive (e.g., Kahneman, 2011; Stanovich, 1999) psychology, where the slow and effortful strategy is often referred to as "analytic", "systematic", or "system 2"

TABLE 5.1 Truth criteria

Criterion	*Analytic evaluation*	*Intuitive evaluation*
Compatibility: Is it compatible with other things I know?	Is this compatible with knowledge retrieved from memory or obtained from trusted sources?	Does this make me stumble or does it flow smoothly?
Coherence: Is it internally coherent?	Do the elements fit together in a logical way? Do the conclusions follow from what is presented?	Does this make me stumble or does it flow smoothly?
Credibility: Does it come from a credible source?	Does the source have the relevant expertise? Does the source have a vested interest? Is the source trustworthy?	Does the source feel familiar and trustworthy?
Consensus: Do other people believe it?	What do my friends say? What do the opinion polls say?	Does it feel familiar?
Evidence: Is there supporting evidence?	Is there supportive evidence in peer-reviewed scientific articles or credible news reports? Do I remember relevant evidence?	Does some evidence easily come to mind?

processing and the fast and intuitive strategy as "intuitive", "heuristic", or "system 1" processing.

Key to intuitive assessments of truth is the ease with which the message can be processed. For example, when something is incompatible with other things we know or the story we are told is incoherent, we stumble and backtrack to make sure we understood it correctly (Johnson-Laird, 2012; Winkielman, Huber, Kavanagh, & Schwarz, 2012). This makes the subjective experience of ease of processing, often referred to as processing fluency, a (fallible) indicator of whether the message may have a problem that needs closer attention. Similar considerations apply to the other truth criteria, as discussed later in the chapter. Throughout, difficult processing marks the message for closer scrutiny, whereas easy processing favors message acceptance.

If ease or difficulty of processing was solely determined by attributes substantively associated with whether a message is likely to be true, relying on one's processing experience would not pose a major problem. However, messages can be easy or difficult to process for many reasons – reading may be slow because the message is incoherent (a relevant criterion) or because the print font is hard to read (which is unrelated to truth). Because people are more sensitive to their subjective experiences than to the source of those experiences (Schwarz, 2012), many incidental influences that have no bearing on the substance of the message can influence its perceived truth. We discuss these incidental influences and their role in media consumption after reviewing the five dominant truth criteria. As will become apparent, when thoughts flow smoothly, people are likely to agree without much critical analysis (see also Oyserman & Dawson, this volume).

The "big five" of truth judgment: analytic and intuitive processes

A claim is more likely to be accepted as true when it is *compatible* with other things one knows than when it is at odds with other knowledge. Compatibility can be assessed analytically by checking the information against one's knowledge, which requires motivation and time (Petty & Cacioppo, 1986). A less demanding indicator is provided by one's metacognitive experiences and affective responses. When something is inconsistent with existing beliefs, people tend to stumble – they take longer to read it, and have trouble processing it (e.g., Taber & Lodge, 2006; Winkielman et al., 2012). Moreover, information that is inconsistent with one's beliefs produces a negative affective response, as shown in research on cognitive consistency (Festinger, 1957; Gawronski & Strack, 2012). Accordingly, one's processing experiences and affective responses can serve as (fallible) indicators of whether a proposition is consistent with other things one believes.

A given claim is also more likely to be accepted as true when it fits a broader story that lends *coherence* to its individual elements, as observed in research on mental models (for a review, see Johnson-Laird, 2012) and analyses of jury decision making (Pennington & Hastie, 1993). Coherence can be determined through a systematic analysis of the relationships between different pieces of declarative information. Alternatively, it can be assessed by attending to one's processing experience: coherent stories are easier to process than stories with internal contradictions (Johnson-Laird, 2012), which makes ease of processing a (fallible) indicator of coherence. Indeed, people draw on their fluency experience when they evaluate how well things "go together" (Topolinski, 2012), as observed in judgments of semantic coherence (Topolinski & Strack, 2008, 2009) and syllogistic reasoning (Morsanyi & Handley, 2012).

Information is also more likely to be accepted as true when it comes from a credible and trustworthy source. As decades of persuasion research illustrates, evaluations of *source credibility* can be based on declarative information that bears, for example, on the communicator's expertise, education, achievement, or institutional affiliation and the presence or absence of conflicting interests (for reviews, see Eagly & Chaiken, 1993; Petty & Cacioppo, 1986). However, credibility judgments can also be based on feelings of familiarity. In daily life, people trust familiar others more than strangers (Luhmann, 1979), from personal interactions to e-commerce (Gefen, 2000). Familiarity resulting from previous encounters or even just repeatedly seeing pictures of a face is sufficient to increase perceptions of honesty and sincerity as well as agreement with what the person says (Brown, Brown, & Zoccoli, 2002; Weisbuch & Mackie, 2009). Similarly, the mere repetition of a name can make an unknown name seem familiar, making its bearer "famous overnight" (Jacoby, Woloshyn, & Kelley, 1989), which may also increase perceived expertise. Familiar people are also easier to recognize and remember, and their names become easier to pronounce with repeated encounters. Variables that influence the ease with which source information can be processed can therefore enhance the perceived credibility of the source. Indeed, a given claim is more likely to be judged true when the name of its source is easy to pronounce (Newman et al., 2014).

To assess the likely truth of a claim, people also consider whether others believe it – if many people agree, there's probably something to it. This *social consensus* (Festinger, 1954) criterion is central to many social influence processes and is sometimes referred to as the principle of "social proof" (Cialdini, 2009). As numerous studies indicated, people are more confident in their beliefs if they are shared by others (Newcomb, 1943; Visser & Mirabile, 2004), more likely to endorse a message if many others have done so as well (Cialdini, 2009), and place more trust in what they remember if others remember it similarly (Harris & Hahn, 2009; Ross, Buehler, & Karr, 1998). Conversely, perceiving dissent reliably undermines message acceptance, which makes reports on real or fabricated controversies an efficient strategy for swaying public opinion (Lewandowsky, Ecker, Seifert, Schwarz, & Cook, 2012; Lewandowsky, Gignac, & Vaughan, 2013). To assess the extent of consensus, people may consult public opinion polls or ask their friends. Alternatively, they may rely on how "familiar" the belief feels – after all, one should have encountered popular beliefs, shared by many, more frequently than unpopular beliefs, held by few. Empirically, familiar information is easier to read, understand, and remember than unfamiliar information, which makes ease of processing a (fallible) indicator of familiarity and popularity. Accordingly, incidental changes in ease of processing can influence perceived consensus.

Finally, people's confidence in a belief increases with the *amount of supporting evidence*. Support can be assessed through an external search, as in a scientific literature review or through recall of pertinent information from memory; in either case, confidence increases with the amount of supportive information. Alternatively, support can be gauged from how easy it is to find supportive evidence – the more evidence there is, the easier it should be to find some (in memory or in the literature). This lay theory is at the heart of Tversky and Kahneman's (1973) availability heuristic. Unfortunately, this heuristic can be misleading. If the only supportive piece of information comes to mind easily because it has been endlessly repeated or is very vivid and memorable, we may erroneously conclude that support is strong. Moreover, attention to *what* comes to mind and attention to the *ease* with which it does so will often lead to different conclusions. On the one hand, reliance on the substantive arguments brought to mind results in higher confidence the more arguments one retrieves or generates. On the other hand, reliance on ease of recall results in lower confidence the more arguments one tries to come up with because finding many arguments is difficult, which suggests that there probably aren't many (Haddock, Rothman, Reber, & Schwarz, 1999; for reviews, see Schwarz, 1998; Schwarz & Vaughn, 2002).

Regardless of which truth criteria people draw on, easily processed information enjoys an advantage over information that is difficult to process: it feels more familiar, more compatible with one's beliefs, more internally consistent, more widely held, better supported, and more likely to have come from a credible source. These inferences reflect that familiar, frequently encountered information and information that is coherent and compatible with one's knowledge is indeed easier to process than information that is not. Hence, ease of processing provides heuristically useful – but fallible – information for assessing how well a claim meets major truth criteria.

Making claims "feel" true

So far, our discussion highlighted that ease or difficulty of processing can result both from variables that are meaningfully related to key criteria of truth or from incidental influences. This is important for two reasons. From a research perspective, it allows researchers to manipulate processing fluency in ways that are independent of substantive characteristics of a message and its source. From an applied perspective, it highlights that claims can "feel" true merely because they are easy to process, which provides many opportunities for manipulation. Next, we review some of the most important variables that influence the ease or difficulty of message processing.

Repetition

Demagogues have known for millennia that truth can be created through frequent repetition of a lie – as Hitler put it, "Propaganda must confine itself to a few points and repeat them over and over again" (cited in Toland, 1976, p. 221). Empirical research supports demagogues' intuition. Studying wartime rumors, Allport and Lepkin (1945) found that the best predictor of whether people believed a rumor was the number of times they were exposed to it. Testing this observation in the laboratory, Hasher, Goldstein, and Toppino (1977) asked participants to rate their confidence that each of 60 statements was true. Some statements were factually correct (e.g., "Lithium is the lightest of all metals"), whereas others were not (e.g., "The People's Republic of China was founded in 1947"). Participants provided their ratings on three occasions, each two weeks apart. Across these sessions, some statements were repeated once or twice, whereas others were not, resulting in one, two, or three exposures. As expected, participants were more confident that a given statement was true the more often they had seen it, independent of whether it was factually true or false. Numerous follow-up studies confirmed the power of repetition across many content domains, from trivia statements (e.g., Bacon, 1979) to marketing claims (e.g., Hawkins & Hoch, 1992) and political beliefs (e.g., Arkes, Hackett, & Boehm, 1989), with the time delay between exposure and judgment ranging from minutes (e.g., Begg & Armour, 1991) to months (Brown & Nix, 1996). Dechêne, Stahl, Hansen, and Wänke (2010) provide a comprehensive meta-analysis of this "illusory truth" effect.

The influence of repetition is most pronounced for claims that people feel uncertain about, but is also observed when more diagnostic information about the claims is available (Fazio, Rand, & Pennycook, 2019; Unkelbach & Greifeneder, 2018). Worse, repetition even increases agreement among people who actually know that the claim is false – if only they thought about it (Fazio, Brashier, Payne, & Marsh, 2015). For example, repeating the statement "The Atlantic Ocean is the largest ocean on Earth" increased its acceptance even among people who knew that the Pacific is larger. When the repeated statement felt familiar, they nodded along without checking it against their knowledge. Even warning people that some of the claims they will be shown are false does not eliminate the effect, although it attenuates its size. More importantly, warnings only attenuate the influence of repetition when they *precede* exposure to the claims – warning people *after* they have seen the claims has no discernable influence (Jalbert, Newman, & Schwarz, 2019).

Repetition also increases perceived social consensus, that is, the perception that a belief is shared by many others. Weaver, Garcia, Schwarz, and Miller (2007) had participants read opinion statements purportedly taken from a group discussion in which a given opinion was presented once or thrice. Each opinion statement was attributed to a group member. Not surprisingly, participants assumed that more people shared the opinion when they read it three times from three different group members (72%) than when they read it only once (57%). However, reading the opinion three times from the *same* group member was almost as influential, resulting in a consensus estimate of 67% – apparently, the single repetitive source sounded like a chorus. Later studies showed that people trust an eyewitness report more the more often it is repeated, even when all repetitions come from the same single witness (Foster, Huthwaite, Yesberg, Garry, & Loftus, 2012). Similarly, newspaper readers are more confident in the accuracy of a report when the same message is presented in several newspapers, even if all newspapers solely rely on the same single interview with the same speaker (Yousif, Aboody, & Keil, 2019). Such findings suggest that frequent repetition of the same soundbite in TV news can give the message a familiarity that increases its perceived popularity and truth. This concern also applies to social media, where the same message keeps showing up as friends and friends of friends like it and repost it, resulting in many exposures within a network.

Beyond repetition

Despite its popularity with past and present demagogues, repetition is just one of many variables that can facilitate easy processing of a statement, making the statement appear more popular, credible, and true. Next, we review some of these other variables.

Reber and Schwarz (1999) manipulated the ease of reading through the *color contrast* of the print font. Depending on condition, some statements (e.g., 'Orsono is a city in Chile') were easy to read due to high color contrast (e.g., dark blue print on a white background), whereas others were difficult to read due to low color contrast (e.g., light blue print on a white background). As predicted, the same statement was more likely to be judged true when it was easy rather than difficult to read. Similarly, the readability of *print fonts* can influence intuitive assessments of truthfulness and the extent to which we closely scrutinize a message. For example, when asked, "How many animals of each kind did Moses take on the Ark?" most people answer "two" even though they know that the biblical actor was Noah, not Moses. Song and Schwarz (2008) presented this Moses question (taken from Erickson & Mattson, 1981) in one of the fonts shown in Figure 5.1. They warned participants that some of the questions may be misleading, in which case they should answer "Can't say". When the Moses question was presented in the easy to read black Arial font, 88% failed to notice a problem and answered "two", whereas only 53% did so when the question was presented in the more difficult to read gray Brush font.

Other variables that influence ease of processing have similar effects. For example, handwritten essays are more compelling when the *handwriting* is easy to read (Greifeneder et al., 2010) and so are spoken messages when the speaker's *accent* is easy to understand (Levy-Ari & Keysar, 2010). Similarly, the same conference talk is less impressive when its video recording has low *audio quality*, and a

Print font	% answering without noticing error
How many animals of each kind did Moses take on the Ark?	88%
How many animals of each kind did Moses take on the Ark?	53%

FIGURE 5.1   Print font and the detection of misleading information

Source: Adapted from Song and Schwarz (2008), Experiment 1.

poor phone connection during a researcher's radio interview can impair listeners' impression of the quality of her research program (Newman & Schwarz, 2018). People also find a statement to be more true when presented with a version of it that *rhymes* rather than one that doesn't, even when the two versions are substantively equivalent (McGlone & Tofighbakhsh, 2000). Even a *photo* without any probative value can increase acceptance of a statement, provided the photo makes it easier to imagine what the statement is about (for a review, see Newman & Zhang, this volume).

Merely having a name that is easy to *pronounce* is sufficient to endow the person with higher credibility and trustworthiness. For example, consumers trust an online seller more when the seller's eBay username is easy to pronounce – they are more likely to believe that the product will live up to the seller's promises and that the seller will honor the advertised return policy (Silva, Chrobot, Newman, Schwarz, & Topolinski, 2017). Similarly, the same claim is more likely to be accepted as true when the name of its source is easy to pronounce (Newman et al., 2014).

As this selective review indicates, any variable that can influence ease of processing can also influence judgments of truth. This is the case because people are very sensitive to their processing experience but insensitive to where this experience comes from. When their attention is directed to the incidental source of their experience, the informational value of the experienced ease or difficulty is undermined and its influence attenuated or eliminated, as predicted by feelings-as-information theory (for reviews, see Schwarz, 2012, 2018).

Analytic versus intuitive processing

As in other domains of judgment, people are more likely to invest the time and effort needed for careful information processing when they are sufficiently motivated and have the time and opportunity to do so (for reviews, see Greifeneder, Bless, & Pham, 2011; Greifeneder & Schwarz, 2014). One may hope that this favors careful processing whenever the issue is important. However, this optimism may not be warranted. In the course of everyday life, messages about issues we consider personally important may reach us when we have other things on our minds and lack the opportunity to engage with them. Over repeated encounters, such messages may become familiar and fluent enough to escape closer scrutiny even when the situation would allow us to engage with them. As reviewed previously, telling recipients that some of the information shown to them is false is only protective when the warning precedes the first exposure; later warnings show little effect (Jalbert et al., 2019). Similarly, the motivation and opportunity to examine a message critically may exert only a limited influence once the message has been encoded (for a review, see Lewandowsky et al., 2012).

Implications for social media

The dynamics of truth judgment have important implications for the acceptance and correction of false information in the real world. Beginning with the proliferation of cable TV and talk radio, citizens in democracies enjoyed ever more opportunities to selectively expose themselves to media that fit their worldview. The advent of social media is the latest step in this development and, in many ways, one might think that social media were designed to make questionable messages seem true. To begin with, most social media messages are short, written in simple language, and presented in optics that are easy to read, which satisfies many of the technical prerequisites for easy processing. These fluent messages are posted by one's friends, a credible source. The content they post is usually compatible with one's own beliefs, given the similarity of opinions and values in friendship networks (for a review of network homophily, see McPherson, Smith-Lovin, & Cook, 2001). Posted messages are liked by other friends, thus confirming social consensus, and reposted, thus ensuring multiple repeated exposures. With each exposure, processing becomes easier and perceptions of social consensus, coherence, and compatibility increase. Comments and related posts provide additional supporting evidence and further enhance familiarity. At the same time, the accumulating likes and reposts ensure that the filtering mechanism of the feed makes exposure to opposing information less and less likely. The *Wall Street Journal*'s "Blue Feed/Red Feed" site illustrates how Facebook's filtering mechanism resulted in profoundly different news feeds for liberals and conservatives during the 2016 elections in the United States, and a growing body of research traces how opinion homophily within networks contributes to controversies between networks (Del Vicario et al., 2016; Gargiulo & Gandica, 2017). The observed narrowing of recipients' information diet on social media is enhanced through the personalization of internet offerings outside of social media, where internet providers and search engines track users' interests to tailor information delivery (Pariser, 2011).

These processes not only increase the acceptance of claims that feel increasingly familiar and compatible with what else one knows but also foster a high sense of expertise and confidence. After all, much of what one sees in one's feed is familiar, which suggests that one knows most of what there is to know about the topic. It has also been seen without much opposing evidence, suggesting that the arguments are undisputed. This enhances what Ross and Ward (1996) described as "naïve realism" – the belief that the world is the way I see it and whoever disagrees is either ill-informed (which motivates persuasion efforts) or ill-intentioned (if persuasion fails). These beliefs further contribute to polarization and the mutual attribution of malevolence.

Implications for the correction of misinformation

That people can arrive at judgments of truth by relying more on analytic or more on intuitive strategies poses a major challenge for public information campaigns aimed at correcting false beliefs. Extensive research in education shows that students' misconceptions can be corrected by confronting them with correct information, showing students step by step why one idea is wrong and another one right, preferably repeating this process multiple times (for reviews, see Vosniadou, 2008). This works best when the recipient wants to acquire the correct information and is sufficiently motivated to pay attention, think through the issues, and remember the new insights (for a review, see Sinatra & Pintrich, 2003). Public information campaigns often follow these procedures by confronting the "myths" with "facts", consistent with content-focused theories of message learning (McQuail, 2000; Rice & Atkin, 2001). While this works in the classroom, with motivated recipients, sufficient time, and the benefit of incentives, the reality of public information campaigns is starkly different. For any given topic, only a small segment of the population will care enough to engage with the details; most are likely to notice the message only in passing, if at all, and will process it superficially while doing something else. Even if they remember the corrective message as intended when tested immediately, it may fade quickly from memory.

Under such conditions, repeating false information in order to correct it may mostly succeed in spreading the false information to disinterested recipients who may otherwise never have encountered it. Not having processed the message in detail, they may now find the false claims a bit more familiar and easier to process when they hear or see them again. This way, the attempt to correct the erroneous beliefs of a few may prepare numerous others to accept those beliefs through repeated exposure (for a review, see Schwarz, Sanna, Skurnik, & Yoon, 2007). For example, Skurnik, Yoon, Park, and Schwarz (2005) exposed older and younger adults once or thrice to product statements like "Shark cartilage is good for your arthritis", and these statements were explicitly marked as "true" or "false". When tested immediately, the corrections seemed successful – all participants were less likely to accept a statement as true the more often they were told that it is false. This is the hoped-for success and most studies stop at this point. But after a three-day delay, repeated warnings backfired and older adults were now more likely to consider a statement "true", the more often they had been explicitly told that it is false. Presumably, the recipients could no longer recall whether the statement had been originally marked as true or false, but still experienced repeated statements as easier to process and more familiar, which made the statements "feel" true.

Even exposing people to only true information can make it more likely that they accept a false version of that information as time passes. Garcia-Marques, Silva, Reber, and Unkelbach (2015) presented participants with ambiguous statements (e.g., "crocodiles sleep with their eyes closed") and later asked them to rate the truth of statements that were either identical to those previously seen or that directly contradicted them (e.g., "crocodiles sleep with their eyes open"). When participants made these judgments immediately, they rated repeated identical statements as more true, and contradicting statements as less true, than novel statements, which they had not seen before. One week later, however, identical as well as contradicting statements seemed more true than novel statements. Put simply, as long as the delay is short enough, people can recall the exact information they just saw and reject the opposite. As time passes, however, the details get lost and contradicting information feels more familiar than information one has never heard of – yes, there was something about crocodiles and their eyes, so that's probably what it was.

As time passes, people may even infer the credibility of the initial source from the confidence with which they hold the belief. For example, Fragale and Heath (2004) exposed participants two or five times to statements like "The wax used to line Cup-o-Noodles cups has been shown to cause cancer in rats". Next, participants learned that some statements were taken from the *National Enquirer* (a low credibility source) and some from *Consumer Reports* (a high credibility source) and had to assign the statements to their likely sources. The more often participants had heard a statement, the more likely they were to attribute it to *Consumer Reports* rather than the *National Enquirer*. In short, frequent exposure not only increases the apparent truth of a statement, it also increases the belief that the statement came from a trustworthy source. Similarly, well-intentioned efforts by the Centers for Disease Control and the *Los Angeles Times* to debunk a rumor about "flesh-eating bananas" morphed into the belief that the *Los Angeles Times* had warned people not to eat those dangerous bananas, thus reinforcing the rumor (Emery, 2000). Such errors in source attribution increase the likelihood that people convey the information to others, who themselves are more likely to accept (and spread) it, given its alleged credible source (Rosnow & Fine, 1976).

Such findings illustrate that attempts to correct misinformation can backfire when they focus solely on message content at the expense of the message's impact on recipients' later processing experience. Even when a corrective message succeeds in changing the beliefs of recipients who deeply care about the topic and process the message with sufficient attention, it may spread the false information to many others who don't care about the topic. Unfortunately, the latter are likely to outnumber the former. In those cases, the successful correction of a few false believers may come at the cost of misleading many bystanders. To avoid such backfire effects, it will usually be safer to refrain from any reiteration of false information and to focus solely on the facts. The more the facts become familiar and fluent, the more likely it is that they will be accepted as true and serve as the basis of judgments and decisions (Lewandowsky et al., 2012; Schwarz et al., 2007, 2016).

Unfortunately, the truth is usually more complicated than false stories, which often involve considerable simplification. This puts the truth at a disadvantage because it is harder to process, understand, and remember. It is therefore important to present true information in ways that facilitate its fluent processing. This requires clear step-by-step exposition and the avoidance of jargon. It also helps to pay close attention to incidental influences on ease of processing. Making the font easy to read and the speaker's pronunciation easy to understand, adding photos and repeating key points are all techniques that should not be left to those who want to mislead – they can also give truth a helping hand and should be used.

Finally, at the individual level, the best protection against the influence of misinformation is skepticism at the time the information is first encountered (for a review, see Lewandowsky et al., 2012). Once people have processed the false information, warnings exert little influence. In addition to explicit warnings, general feelings of suspicion and distrust increase message scrutiny and decrease message acceptance (for reviews, see Mayo, 2017; Schwarz & Lee, 2019). Explicit warnings as well as suspicion and distrust entail that the communicator may not adhere to the norms of cooperative conversational conduct (Grice, 1975), thus flagging the message for closer scrutiny. Unfortunately, in a polarized public opinion climate, merely realizing that a message supports the "other" side is itself likely to elicit suspicion and distrust, further impairing correction attempts in polarized contexts.

Acknowledgments

Preparation of this chapter was supported by the Linnie and Michael Katz Endowed Research Fellowship Fund through a fellowship to the second author and funds of the USC Dornsife Mind and Society Center to the first author.

References

Allport, F. H., & Lepkin, M. (1945). Wartime rumors of waste and special privilege: Why some people believe them. *Journal of Abnormal and Social Psychology, 40*, 3–36.

Arkes, H. R., Hackett, C., & Boehm, L. (1989). The generality of the relation between familiarity and judged validity. *Journal of Behavioral Decision Making, 2*, 81–94.

Bacon, F. T. (1979). Credibility of repeated statements: Memory for trivia. *Journal of Experimental Psychology: Human Learning and Memory, 5*, 241–252.

Begg, I., & Armour, V. (1991). Repetition and the ring of truth: Biasing comments. *Canadian Journal of Behavioural Science, 23*, 195–213.

Brown, A. S., Brown, L. A., & Zoccoli, S. L. (2002). Repetition-based credibility enhancement of unfamiliar faces. *The American Journal of Psychology, 115*, 199–2009.

Brown, A. S., & Nix, L. A. (1996). Turning lies into truths: Referential validation of falsehoods. *Journal of Experimental Psychology: Learning, Memory, and Cognition, 22,* 1088–1100.

Cialdini, R. B. (2009). *Influence: Science and practice.* Boston: Pearson Education.

Dechêne, A., Stahl, C., Hansen, J., & Wänke, M. (2010). The truth about the truth: A meta-analytic review of the truth effect. *Personality and Social Psychology Review, 14,* 238–257.

Del Vicario, M., Bessi, A., Zollo, F., Petroni, F., Scala, A., Caldarelli, G., . . . Quattrociocchi, W. (2016). The spreading of misinformation online. *Proceedings of the National Academy of Sciences, 113*(3), 554–559.

Eagly, A. H., & Chaiken, S. (1993). *The psychology of attitudes.* Fort Worth, TX: Harcourt Brace.

Emery, D. (2000, February 23). The great banana scare of 2000. Retrieved May 24, 2002, from http://urbanlegends.about.com/library/weekly/aa022302a.htm

Erickson, T. D., & Mattson, M. E. (1981). From words to meaning: A semantic illusion. *Journal of Verbal Learning & Verbal Behavior, 20,* 540–551.

Fazio, L. K., Brashier, N. M., Payne, B. K., & Marsh, E. J. (2015). Knowledge does not protect against illusory truth. *Journal of Experimental Psychology: General, 144*(5), 993–1002.

Fazio, L. K., Rand, D. G., & Pennycook, G. (2019). Repetition increases perceived truth equally for plausible and implausible statements. *Psychonomic Bulletin & Review, 26*(5), 1705–1710.

Festinger, L. (1954). A theory of social comparison processes. *Human Relations, 7,* 123–146.

Festinger, L. (1957). *A theory of cognitive dissonance.* Evanston, IL: Row, Peterson.

Foster, J. L., Huthwaite, T., Yesberg, J. A., Garry, M., & Loftus, E. (2012). Repetition, not number of sources, increases both susceptibility to misinformation and confidence in the accuracy of eyewitnesses. *Acta Psychologica, 139,* 320–326.

Fragale, A. R., & Heath, C. (2004). Evolving information credentials: The (mis)attribution of believable facts to credible sources. *Personality and Social Psychology Bulletin, 30,* 225–236.

Gabielkov, M., Ramachandran, A., Chaintreau, A., & Legout, A. (2016). Social clicks: What and who gets read on Twitter? *ACM SIGMETRICS Performance Evaluation Review, 44,* 179–192. http://dx.doi.org/10.1145/2896377.2901462

Garcia-Marques, T., Silva, R. R., Reber, R., & Unkelbach, C. (2015). Hearing a statement now and believing the opposite later. *Journal of Experimental Social Psychology, 56,* 126–129.

Gargiulo, F., & Gandica, Y. (2017). The role of homophily in the emergence of opinion controversies. *Journal of Artificial Societies and Social Simulation, 20*(3), 8. doi: 10.18564/jasss.3448. Retrieved from http://jasss.soc.surrey.ac.uk/20/3/8.htm

Gawronski, B., & Strack, F. (Eds.). (2012). *Cognitive consistency: A fundamental principle in social cognition.* New York: Guilford Press.

Gefen, D. (2000). E-commerce: The role of familiarity and trust. *Omega, 28,* 725–737.

Gilbert, D. T. (1991). How mental systems believe. *American Psychologist, 46,* 107–119.

Greifeneder, R., Alt, A., Bottenberg, K., Seele, T., Zelt, S., & Wagener, D. (2010). On writing legibly: Processing fluency systematically biases evaluations of handwritten material. *Social Psychological and Personality Science, 1,* 230–237.

Greifeneder, R., Bless, H., & Pham, M. T. (2011). When do people rely on cognitive and affective feelings in judgment? A review. *Personality and Social Psychology Review, 15,* 107–141.

Greifeneder, R., & Schwarz, N. (2014). Metacognitive processes and subjective experience. In J. W. Sherman, B. Gawronski, & Y. Trope (Eds.), *Dual-process theories of the social mind* (pp. 314–327). New York, NY: Guilford Press.

Grice, H. P. (1975). Logic and conversation. In P. Cole & J. L. Morgan (Eds.), *Syntax and semantics, vol. 3: Speech acts* (pp. 41–58). New York: Academic Press.

Haddock, G., Rothman, A. J., Reber, R., & Schwarz, N. (1999). Forming judgments of attitude certainty, importance, and intensity: The role of subjective experiences. *Personality and Social Psychology Bulletin, 25,* 771–782.

Harris, A. J. L., & Hahn, U. (2009). Bayesian rationality in evaluating multiple testimonies: Incorporating the role of coherence. *Journal of Experimental Psychology: Learning, Memory, and Cognition, 35,* 1366–1372.

Hasher, L., Goldstein, D., & Toppino, T. (1977). Frequency and the conference of referential validity. *Journal of Verbal Learning & Verbal Behavior, 16,* 107–112.

Hasson, U., Simmons, J. P., & Todorov, A. (2005). Believe it or not: On the possibility of suspending belief. *Psychological Science, 16,* 566–571.

Hawkins, S. A., & Hoch, S. J. (1992). Low-involvement learning: Memory without evaluation. *Journal of Consumer Research, 19,* 212–225.

Jacoby, L. L., Woloshyn, V., & Kelley, C. M. (1989). Becoming famous without being recognized: Unconscious influences of memory produced by dividing attention. *Journal of Experimental Psychology: General, 118,* 115–125.

Jalbert, M., Newman, E. J., & Schwarz, N. (2019). *Only half of what I tell you is true: How experimental procedures lead to an underestimation of the truth effect.* Manuscript under review.

Johnson-Laird, P. N. (2012). Mental models and consistency. In B. Gawronski & F. Strack (Eds.), *Cognitive consistency: A fundamental principle in social cognition* (pp. 225–243). New York: Guilford Press.

Kahneman, D. (2011). *Thinking, fast and slow.* New York: Macmillan.

Levy-Ari, S., & Keysar, B. (2010). Why don't we believe non-native speakers? The influence of accent on credibility. *Journal of Experimental Social Psychology, 46,* 1093–1096.

Lewandowsky, S., Ecker, U. K. H., Seifert, C., Schwarz, N., & Cook, J. (2012). Misinformation and its correction: Continued influence and successful debiasing. *Psychological Science in the Public Interest, 13,* 106–131.

Lewandowsky, S., Gignac, G. E., & Vaughan, S. (2013). The pivotal role of perceived scientific consensus in acceptance of science. *Nature Climate Change, 3,* 399–404.

Luhmann, N. (1979). *Trust and power.* Chichester, UK: Wiley.

Mayo, R. (2017). Cognition is a matter of trust: Distrust tunes cognitive processes. *European Review of Social Psychology, 26,* 283–327.

McGlone, M. S., & Tofighbakhsh, J. (2000). Birds of a feather flock conjointly (?): Rhyme as reason in aphorisms. *Psychological Science, 11,* 424–428.

McPherson, M., Smith-Lovin, L., & Cook. J. M. (2001). Birds of a feather: Homophily in social networks. *Annual Review of Sociology, 27,* 415–444.

McQuail, D. (2000). *McQuail's mass communication theory.* Newbury Park, CA: Sage Publications.

Morsanyi, K., & Handley, S. J. (2012). Logic feels so good: I like it! Evidence for intuitive detection of logicality in syllogistic reasoning. *Journal of Experimental Psychology: Learning, Memory, and Cognition, 38,* 596–616.

Newcomb, T. M. (1943). *Personality and social change.* New York: Holt, Rinehart, & Winston.

Newman, E. J., Sanson, M., Miller, E. K., Quigley-McBride, A., Foster, J. L., Bernstein, D. M., & Garry, M. (2014). People with easier to pronounce names promote truthiness of claims. *PLoS One, 9*(2). doi: 10.1371/journal.pone.0088671

Newman, E. J., & Schwarz, N. (2018). Good sound, good research: How audio quality influences perceptions of the researcher and research. *Science Communication, 40*(2), 246–257.

Newman, E. J., & Zhang, L. (2020). Truthiness: How nonprobative photos shape beliefs. In R. Greifeneder, M. Jaffé, E. J. Newman, & N. Schwarz (Eds.), *The psychology of fake news: Accepting, sharing, and correcting misinformation* (pp. 90–114). London, UK: Routledge.

Oyserman, D., & Dawson, A. (2020). Your fake news, our fakes: Identity-based motivation shapes what we believe, share, and accept. In R. Greifeneder, M. Jaffé, E. J. Newman, & N. Schwarz (Eds.), *The psychology of fake news: Accepting, sharing, and correcting misinformation* (pp. 173–195). London, UK: Routledge.

Pariser, E. (2011). *The filter bubble: How the new personalized web is changing what we read and how the think.* New York: Penguin Books.

Pennington, N., & Hastie, R. (1993). The story model for juror decision making. In R. Hastie (Ed.), *Inside the juror* (pp. 192–223). New York: Cambridge University Press.

Petty, R. E., & Cacioppo, J. T. (1986). The elaboration likelihood model of persuasion. *Advances in Experimental Social Psychology, 19,* 123–205.

Reber, R., & Schwarz, N. (1999). Effects of perceptual fluency on judgments of truth. *Consciousness and Cognition, 8,* 338–342.

Rice, R., & Atkin, C. (Eds.). (2001). *Public communication campaigns* (3rd ed.). Newbury Park, CA: Sage Publications.

Rosnow, R. L., & Fine, G. A. (1976). *Rumor and gossip: The social psychology of hearsay.* New York: Elsevier.

Ross, L., & Ward, A. (1996). Naive realism in everyday life: Implications for social conflict and misunderstanding. In E. S. Reed, E. Turiel, & T. Brown (Eds.), *Values and knowledge* (pp. 103–135). Hillsdale, NJ: Lawrence Erlbaum.

Ross, M., Buehler, R., & Karr, J. W. (1998). Assessing the accuracy of conflicting autobiographical memories. *Memory and Cognition, 26,* 1233–1244.

Schul, Y., Mayo, R., & Burnstein, E. (2008). The value of distrust. *Journal of Experimental Social Psychology, 44,* 1293–1302.

Schwarz, N. (1994). Judgment in a social context: Biases, shortcomings, and the logic of conversation. *Advances in Experimental Social Psychology, 26,* 123–162.

Schwarz, N. (1996). *Cognition and communication: Judgmental biases, research methods, and the logic of conversation.* Hillsdale, NJ: Erlbaum.

Schwarz, N. (1998). Accessible content and accessibility experiences: The interplay of declarative and experiential information in judgment. *Personality and Social Psychology Review, 2,* 87–99.

Schwarz, N. (2012). Feelings-as-information theory. In P. A. Van Lange, A. W. Kruglanski, & E. Higgins (Eds.), *Handbook of theories of social psychology* (pp. 289–308). Thousand Oaks, CA: Sage Publications.

Schwarz, N. (2015). Metacognition. In M. Mikulincer, P. R. Shaver, E. Borgida, & J. A. Bargh (Eds.), *APA handbook of personality and social psychology: Attitudes and social cognition* (pp. 203–229). Washington, DC: APA.

Schwarz, N. (2018). Of fluency, beauty, and truth: Inferences from metacognitive experiences. In J. Proust & M. Fortier (Eds.), *Metacognitive diversity: An interdisciplinary approach* (pp. 25–46). New York: Oxford University Press.

Schwarz, N., & Lee, S. W. S. (2019). The smell of suspicion: How the nose curbs gullibility. In J. P. Forgas & R. F. Baumeister (Eds.), *The social psychology of gullibility: Fake news, conspiracy theories, and irrational beliefs* (pp. 234–252). New York: Routledge and Psychology Press.

Schwarz, N., Newman, E., & Leach, W. (2016). Making the truth stick and the myths fade: Lessons from cognitive psychology. *Behavioral Science & Policy, 2*(1), 85–95.

Schwarz, N., Sanna, L. J., Skurnik, I., & Yoon, C. (2007). Metacognitive experiences and the intricacies of setting people straight: Implications for debiasing and public information campaigns. *Advances in Experimental Social Psychology*, *39*, 127–161.

Schwarz, N., & Vaughn, L. A. (2002). The availability heuristic revisited: Ease of recall and content of recall as distinct sources of information. In T. Gilovich, D. Griffin, & D. Kahneman (Eds.), *Heuristics and biases: The psychology of intuitive judgment* (pp. 103–119). Cambridge: Cambridge University Press.

Silva, R. R., Chrobot, N., Newman, E., Schwarz, N., & Topolinski, S. (2017). Make it short and easy: Username complexity determines trustworthiness above and beyond objective reputation. *Frontiers in Psychology*, *8*, 2200.

Sinatra, G. M., & Pintrich, P. (2003). The role of intentions in conceptual change learning. In G. M. Sinatra & P. R. Pintrich (Eds.), *Intentional conceptual change*. Mahwah, NJ: Lawrence Erlbaum Associates.

Skurnik, I., Yoon, C., Park, D. C., & Schwarz, N. (2005). How warnings about false claims become recommendations. *Journal of Consumer Research*, *31*, 713–724.

Song, H., & Schwarz, N. (2008). Fluency and the detection of misleading questions: Low processing fluency attenuates the Moses illusion. *Social Cognition*, *26*, 791–799.

Sperber, D., & Wilson, D. (1986). *Relevance: Communication and cognition*. Cambridge, MA: Harvard University Press.

Stanovich, K. E. (1999). *Who is rational? Studies of individual differences in reasoning*. Mahwah: Erlbaum.

Taber, C. S., & Lodge, M. (2006). Motivated skepticism in the evaluation of political beliefs. *American Journal of Political Science*, *50*(3), 755–769.

Toland, J. (1976). *Adolf Hitler*. Garden City, NY: Doubleday.

Topolinski, S. (2012). Nonpropositional consistency. In B. Gawronski & F. Strack (Eds.), *Cognitive consistency: A fundamental principle in social cognition* (pp. 112–131). New York: Guilford Press.

Topolinski, S., & Strack, F. (2008). Where there's a will: There's no intuition: The unintentional basis of semantic coherence judgments. *Journal of Memory and Language*, *58*, 1032–1048.

Topolinski, S., & Strack, F. (2009). The architecture of intuition: Fluency and affect determine intuitive judgments of semantic and visual coherence and judgments of grammaticality in artificial grammar learning. *Journal of Experimental Psychology: General*, *138*, 39–63.

Tversky, A., & Kahneman, D. (1973). Availability: A heuristic for judging frequency and probability. *Cognitive Psychology*, *5*, 207–232.

Unkelbach, C., & Greifeneder, R. (2018). Experiential fluency and declarative advice jointly inform judgments of truth. *Journal of Experimental Social Psychology*, *79*, 78–86.

Visser, P. S., & Mirabile, R. R. (2004). Attitudes in the social context: The impact of social network composition on individual-level attitude strength. *Journal of Personality and Social Psychology*, *87*, 779–795.

Vosniadou, S. (Ed.). (2008). *International handbook of research on conceptual change*. New York, NY: Routledge.

Weaver, K., Garcia, S. M., Schwarz, N., & Miller, D. T. (2007). Inferring the popularity of an opinion from its familiarity: A repetitive voice can sound like a chorus. *Journal of Personality and Social Psychology*, *92*, 821–833.

Weisbuch, M., & Mackie, D. (2009). False fame, perceptual clarity, or persuasion? Flexible fluency attribution in spokesperson familiarity effects. *Journal of Consumer Psychology*, *19*(1), 62–72.

Winkielman, P., Huber, D. E., Kavanagh, L., & Schwarz, N. (2012). Fluency of consistency: When thoughts fit nicely and flow smoothly. In B. Gawronski & F. Strack (Eds.), *Cognitive consistency: A fundamental principle in social cognition* (pp. 89–111). New York: Guilford Press.

Yousif, S. R., Aboody, R., & Keil, F. C. (2019). The illusion of consensus: A failure to distinguish between true and false consensus. *Psychological Science, 30*(8), 1195–1204.

2

CONNECTIONS

Ciarán Mc Mahon

After setting up their profile, users' second task after creating a social media account is probably connecting with other users. From friends to followers, social media is, for many people, largely about publicly connecting with each other.

It gives ordinary people access to potentially huge audiences –for free and at the click of few buttons. But is it all really that easy? And how real are our audiences? How much work do we have to put into building our connections – and what price do we pay to access them? The critical point is to weigh up the benefits and drawbacks of being able to connect to so many different people in one particular place.

CASE STUDY: THE ICE BUCKET CHALLENGE

The 'ice bucket challenge' is often described as one of social media's greatest successes. It began with a silly prank, but it raised a serious amount of money for a worthy cause. While it is genuinely difficult to carry out accurate historical research on social media services,[1] it seems that an ice bucket challenge existed on Facebook for some time before it became so very popular.[2] The format was there from the start – a video posted to Facebook of someone stating that they have accepted the challenge, and then getting a bucket of ice poured over their head. After some shrieking, the victim calls on some of their social media connections to do the same within 24 hours or donate to a particular charity as a forfeit.

It only became associated with the disease known as Amyotrophic Lateral Sclerosis (also known as Lou Gehrig's Disease) when Chris Kennedy, from Sarasota, Florida, was given the challenge by a friend.[3] He selected the Amyotrophic Lateral Sclerosis Association as his charity of choice and nominated a relative of his, whose partner was suffering from the disease, to take the challenge. From there it spread through his extended family and friends, but also through supporters of the ALS Association, many of whom put in a huge effort to spread the challenge through their personal networks. The Association itself reportedly began seeing an unusual surge in donations by the end of July, and before long the challenge was being issued to all manner of celebrities, including Mark Zuckerberg.

While some analysts have argued that not everyone who made a video donated, I think this misses the point. The logic of the challenges is that the people 'called out' in the video must dunk themselves within 24 hours or donate as a forfeit. If you're too busy to make a video, or afraid of ice-cold water, you can get out of it by simply opening your wallet. That's the premise of the challenge. So really, if you actually did pour a bucket of ice over yourself, you shouldn't have to donate. But, of course, that isn't what happened.

It seems that the 'feel-good' quality of videos spreading through social media connections meant that the logic of the forfeit was forgotten as the phenomenon took off. People who dunked themselves donated money, and, more than likely, lots of people who weren't challenged at all donated money too.

By the beginning of September 2014, over 17 million videos related to the ice bucket challenge had been posted to Facebook, which had apparently been viewed by more than 440 million people.[4] Of course, as the summer drew to an end, and the idea of soaking oneself in ice-cold water became less appealing, this dropped off drastically. However, the phenomenon resulted in the Amyotrophic Lateral Sclerosis Association receiving over $100 million in additional funding, which was put towards research which ultimately found a breakthrough[5] in the study of the disease. This does not include many other charities who also raised significant amounts of money. As a result, the ice bucket challenge became the blueprint for countless more 'challenges', where many other charities and causes would also seek to harness the power of social media connections.

BONDING AND BRIDGING

But outside of such cultural phenomena, what do we gain from adding people on social media, some of whom we probably don't know very well? The answer to these questions means talking about resources and support.

One of social media's most highly cited research papers was published at Michigan State University in 2007. In this study,[6] Ellison, Steinfield and Lampe were interested in how using Facebook might interact with users' psychological well-being, specifically in a concept called 'social capital'. This refers to the observation that as we know more or less people, we gain or lose valuable information and opportunities. Social scientists generally work on the basis of there being two types of social capital: bonding and bridging. The former refers to the type of resources one gains from close relationships, such as family and best friends: people who would do literally anything for you. And the latter refers to the type of things gained from casual acquaintances: people who might give you information, but probably not emotional support. As such, while bonding social capital is much more valuable than bridging, generally speaking we have fewer connections that produce the former than the latter.

The researchers asked participants several questions regarding their Facebook behaviours, such as how many Facebook friends they had and how many minutes they thought they had spent on Facebook in the last month. But they were also asked whether or not they agreed with attitude statements like 'I am proud to tell people I'm on Facebook', 'I feel out of touch when I haven't logged onto Facebook for a while' and 'I would be sorry if Facebook shut down'. Collated together, participants' responses to all these items were used as a measure of the 'intensity' of their Facebook usage.

What Ellison and colleagues found was that this 'Facebook usage intensity' was strongly associated with both creating and maintaining bridging social capital. However, it was only weakly associated with bonding social capital. So, for example, you might have met someone once a few years ago and added them on Facebook but have no real desire to ever meet them again. Then one day, they post a social media update with job advertisement you're interested in. This is the kind of resource that you wouldn't have if you didn't have that Facebook connection. But, on the other hand, with regards to creating deeper, more meaningful relationships, this paper doesn't show that being connected on Facebook is much use.

So, to go back to the ice bucket challenge – you probably won't call out someone with whom you only have a bridging social capital kind of relationship. You might like their video, and they might like yours, but you will probably reserve your nominations for the sort of people with whom you have a bonding social capital kind of relationship.

Interestingly, these associations were only found with regards to Facebook usage intensity – they were not found with regards to internet use. You have to be interacting with people online – for example, on social media like Facebook – to accumulate social capital. As such, it is pretty easy to see how Facebook is very useful to the type of person that Ellison and her team were surveying. It allows college students to cheaply maintain friendships with their high school friends back home, and it also allows them to connect with new classmates – all in all, a very neat psychological tool.

But is it always this simple? And have things changed since 2007? A more recent paper[7] by researchers at the University of the West of England is revealing in this regard. These researchers were also interested in social capital, but in relation to the newer social media service, Snapchat. Like Ellison and her team in 2007, in 2016 Piwek and Joinson carried out a survey of users. However, they noted that the 'transient nature' of Snapchat presents certain methodological difficulties. Bear in mind that the whole point of Snapchat is that its images are supposed to vanish once viewed by the intended recipient. So how do you study that?

Consequently, unlike in the study mentioned earlier, where participants were asked about their overall Facebook usage, in this study participants were asked to focus on the most recent Snap that they had received. In other respects, Piwek and Joinson carried out a similar study to Ellison and co-workers. It also used a college student population, and they adapted the 'Facebook intensity scale' to measure the intensity of Snapchat usage, using largely identical questions. This adaptation of measures across studies is useful as it allows us to validly compare their results.

Strikingly, in direct contrast to Ellison's Facebook study, Piwek and Johnson found that Snapchat usage was associated with bonding social capital, but less so with bridging social capital. In other words, Snapchat seems to be most useful in the context of deep and meaningful relationships, rather than casual acquaintances. The authors suggest that this is due to a number of factors. For one thing, they note that their participants reported using Snapchat to communicate with a small number of friends – certainly a far smaller number than one would expect on Facebook. For another, Piwek and Joinson also suggest that Snapchat offers a more intimate and more private conversational setting than does Facebook. Hence, once again, we can see that different social media services can offer different psychological experiences to their users in how they connect with each other.

As an aside, this study was carried out before the Snapchat 'Snapstreak' feature became popular. In the new version of Snapchat launched in March 2016,[8] if users sent each other Snaps every day, they were rewarded with a fire symbol beside their friend's name, and a number representing the amount of days they kept this interaction going. Consequently, with this sort of 'gamification' of its social media service, Snapchat encouraged the development of close friendships that would create this kind of bonding social capital. But how many people can you actually keep this level of interaction up with? Let me tell you a curious tale about groups of gorillas and the size of their skulls.

CLIQUES AND CONTEXTS

The quantity of people we connect with on social media brings us to one of the more famous concepts in evolutionary psychology. In 1992, anthropologist Robin Dunbar wrote an influential paper[9] on brain sizes in humanity's nearest relatives. The purpose of this study was to examine the possibility of a correlation between the size of primates' neocortexes and the size of their social groups. Remarkably, Dunbar showed that, indeed, primates like lemurs do have both smaller brains and smaller social groups than, for example, gorillas, who have both bigger brains and bigger social groups. This is known as the 'social brain hypothesis' and while it is not a watertight law – it isn't accurate for orangutans, for example, who seem to live in smaller groups than their brain size would imply – it stands to reason that one might extrapolate from this trend to ourselves. How big should human social groups be, given the size of our brains? According to Dunbar, the answer seems to be around 150. Admittedly this is an average, for what he termed our 'egocentric social network', but it did become henceforth known as 'Dunbar's number'.

The idea of natural human social group sizes is an interesting finding for psychology generally, but even more so for social media research, which became very interested in the 150 number. However, in later work, Dunbar showed how human networks also include a 'sympathy group' of about 15 individuals, as well as a 'support clique' of five individuals. The larger group is defined as the sort of people you would describe as close friends, who you would contact at least once a month, whereas the smaller group are those who you would rely on for emotional support. So it is a simplification to talk about 'Dunbar's number' on social media connections, as if there is only one – there are two more that we should be looking for too.

The core issue here is how our apparent neurological limits are improved by the affordances of social media. Does social media allow us to be more time-efficient with our connections? Recently, Dunbar has tackled this issue head on in a 2016 paper with two surveys of several thousand UK adults.[10]

Dunbar did indeed find that most of his participant's personal social networks contained roughly 150 individuals, and, within that, many did indeed have a sympathy group of about 15 individuals, as well as a support clique of about five. But what is rather striking is that these numbers were largely unaffected by how many social media connections participants had. In other words, connecting with lots of people did not help social media users gain more close friendships – the sympathy groups and support cliques stayed roughly the same size.

As such, Dunbar shows that, despite the fact that social media makes it easier to connect with lots of people, that doesn't mean we can therefore gain more emotional support. Meaningfully connecting with people still takes time.

Notably, while there doesn't seem to be much research combining the 'social capital' concept mentioned previously with Dunbar's numbers, these findings do seem to make sense together: social media may help you increase the quantity of your connections, but not necessarily the quality. One last thing that Dunbar points out is worth noting here. Social media services allow us to gather our connections in the one place, but they don't generally let us organise them into a hierarchy of importance of the kind he is interested in.

But perhaps we might not want to do that publicly. In bygone days on Myspace, users agonised over which of their connections to put in their 'Top 8' group of people they wanted to visibly list on their profile as friends. That leads us to another aspect of connecting with lots of people on social media. Psychology is not only interested in how we cope with this *neurologically*, but also how we manage it *socially*.

A potential drawback of social media is that users might want to segment their connections into different groups. For example, you may not have any problem with being connected to your boss on LinkedIn but might feel differently if they sent you a Facebook Friend request. Keeping walls between our social media connections like this is a fairly normal desire, but it is a pretty difficult one to achieve. In practice, these walls don't hold, because, as Marwick and boyd say, 'context collapse' occurs between them.[11]

Their 2010 paper involved an interesting methodology: asking Twitter users, on Twitter, about who their tweets were written for. That's a critical problem with communicating on social media: despite having lots of connections, we don't really have much certainty about who is paying attention to us at any given time. As such, Marwick and boyd use the concept of the *imagined audience*. Even in everyday conversations, we cannot be exactly sure of how our message will be relayed, or who is listening in on us, but this issue is intensified on social media. When you think about how many of your Twitter followers might be online, who they might retweet to, and under what searches you might appear in, you really have difficulty in imagining who is actually reading your tweets.

Marwick and boyd's survey participants gave some interesting answers to questions about who they were tweeting for. Harking back to Chapter 2 and our talk about identities, it is interesting that several participants stated that their tweets were written for an audience that you might not have considered: they said they were writing for themselves. As Marwick and boyd put it, "consciously speaking to an audience is perceived as inauthentic". Perhaps this was more of a feature of Twitter in 2010, but it is still curious that the first person some social media users trying to connect with is themselves.

Other Twitter users, especially those with large numbers of followers, thought about their audience in terms of fans, as a community, as broadcasting or as consistent political messaging. But even in those contexts, and also users with fewer followers, a common theme emerged: not being able to segment audiences and hence having to aim for a 'lowest common denominator' sort of message – safe, bland and inoffensive.

Marwick and boyd interpreted their survey responses as reflecting either one of two tactics to negotiate these problems. On one hand, some Twitter users simply avoided discussing certain topics altogether – they self-censored for fear of possibly insulting some of their followers. And on the other hand, some Twitter users try to balance their more professional tweets with updates with more personal information. In other words, Twitter users try to avoid annoying their imagined audiences by appearing more human and more relatable. This latter tactic is interesting as it harks back, yet again, to the ongoing difficulty we have on social media in trying to appear authentic. Hence, what Marwick and boyd's paper shows is that while we know that social media services, such as Twitter, create many new opportunities for connection, they also create new tensions and indeed, conflicts.

CONNECTIONS AND CONFLICT

Reflecting on our social media connections as a whole, it is interesting to think about the inter-relationships between them. Besides being our own friends, some of our connections may be connected to each other, some may harass us and some may stay quiet altogether. What do we know about the psychology of them?

For example, when talking about social media in the context of children and parenting, a common fear is the risk of cyberbullying. While previous research focussed on individual and psychological factors associated with this type of aggression, few have examined more social and structural factors. In other words, can we explain why someone is a cyberbully entirely because of their personality, age or gender, or should we also examine their position within the cliques and friendship groups of their school? In that light, a study[12] on how aggressive schoolchildren have unique positions within their social networks is worth teasing out. This paper is noteworthy as it demonstrates the importance of a distinction made in Chapter 1. Because they were interested in social networks *per se*, and in actual fact did not explicitly treat any online services, you could argue that I should not include it in a book on social media at all! But it is very revealing of how little we understand of the psychology of social media connections.

In this study, Festl and Quandt carried out what might be termed a fairly standard social science methodology in an educational context – they gave German high school students a questionnaire to fill in. Like many such research projects, they asked participants questions about their individual characteristics, such as their age, gender, personality traits, how much they used computers and whether or not they were involved in cyberbullying. More unusually, they also asked structural questions, such as asking students to list their best friends. This information allowed the researchers to understand the social network of the school, revealing cliques of friendships, relative levels of popularity and reciprocal relationships. In other words, some students were on a lot more best friends lists than others were.

More crucially, this structural data revealed many interesting findings with regard to cyberbullying. Beyond the individual factors, such as female adolescents being more likely to be the victims of cyberbullying than males, the structural factors revealed some unexpected findings. While both perpetrators and victims of cyberbullying were found to be, in general, less popular than their fellow classmates, this did not hold true for another important category. Those students who had experienced both being the perpetrator and as well as the victim of cyberbullying were highly popular among their classmates. In other words, children who had been a cyberbully, but had also suffered cyberbullying themselves, were more popular than children who had only been cyberbullies, or only been victims.

Fascinatingly, Festl and Quandt also say that, while not statistically significant, it seems that these 'perpetrator/victims' showed a curious pattern of connection within the social network as a whole. A visual representation of the participants' structural relationships revealed that perpetrator/victims were often found to be links between different cliques, rather than central to any clique. This position seems to give them a certain amount of influence over distinct groups, but also vulnerable to being attacked by either. As such, when we examined how aggression like cyberbullying occurs online, it seems that we have a lot yet to learn about the psychology of social media connections. Festl and Quandt conclude rather bluntly that, without taking these kinds of structural factors into account, explanations for online aggression like cyberbullying will remain insufficient.

However, this is in reference to social connections where there is some level of actual interaction. You would be forgiven for thinking that there is nothing interesting happening in our social media connections where there are is no interaction at all. But there is, and the research here is quite revealing of the psychology of these services: welcome to the wonderful world of FOMO. An early paper on this topic by Przybylski and colleagues continues to set the agenda here, as it developed a questionnaire to measure 'fear of missing out', and tested it over three studies.[13] The final version of this scale included such items as "When I go on vacation, I continue to keep tabs on what my friends are doing". Przybylski and colleagues were interested in understanding how fear of missing out correlated with other psychological issues, namely its motivational, emotional and behavioural associations. What they found was that FOMO is primarily experienced by young people, and by young men more than young women. It is also associated with not being psychologically satisfied in a number of areas, including personal autonomy, relatedness and competence. In other words, if you feel like you lack independence, closeness to other people and general capability, you are probably at risk of experiencing FOMO when you go on social media. Again, doesn't this strike you as being similar to the deeper challenge of social media: the struggle to be authentic?

Hence, it would probably be a good idea to think twice before we post content on social media – even if it is positive or jolly, we have no idea how it may make our connections feel. In particular, those people who are struggling to find their place in the world may find our apparently perfect lives difficult to stomach. But we will be talking more about updates in the next chapter.

SUMMARY

In this chapter we saw how social media connections can be valuable, though not in the most straightforward manner. While the ice bucket challenge supports the core social media value that connecting with people is a good thing, in personal circumstances, things are more complex. We saw that Facebook helped college students create and maintain connections with acquaintances – but wasn't much help for closer relationships. Yet the opposite was true with Snapchat, which is better for maintaining close friendships than associates. You have to pick your social media service to suit your relationships.

Regarding our connections as a whole, we discussed 'Dunbar's number', which suggested a neurological limit to the size of our social groups. Not only was it reflected in our social media connections, but so were the sympathy group and the support clique – indicating that we are only able to emotionally connect with a certain number of people, whether online or not.

Furthermore, we have the issue of context collapse – not wanting everyone to see every update we post, but having no idea who is paying attention. So we only share updates that won't offend anyone, or balance with personal revelations, in order to appear more relatable to our 'imagined audience'.

We also considered the friction that can occur between our connections. Notably, perpetrators and victims of cyberbullying do not seem to be popular within their schoolyard social networks, but perpetrator/victims seem to be particularly socially influential. Finally, we muse about that quiet spot in our social media connections, those people who do not interact, and how we might try to avoid giving them the 'fear of missing out', by being careful about what we put in our updates.

NOTES

1 Levin, J. (2014, August 22). Who invented the ice bucket challenge? *Slate*. Retrieved from www.slate.com/articles/technology/technology/2014/08/who_invented_the_ice_bucket_challenge_a_slate_investigation.single.html

2 Sifferlin, A. (2014, August 18). Here's how the ALS ice bucket challenge actually started. TIME. Retrieved from http://time.com/3136507/als-ice-bucket-challenge-started/

3 van Ogtrop, K. (n.d.). Ever wonder how the whole "Ice Bucket Challenge" started? *Real Simple*. Retrieved from www.realsimple.com/magazine-more/jeanette-senerchia-ice-bucket

4 Facebook. (2014, August 18). The ice bucket challenge on Facebook. *Facebook Newsroom*. Retrieved from https://newsroom.fb.com/news/2014/08/the-ice-bucket-challenge-on-facebook/

5 Woolf, N. (2016, July 27). Remember the ice bucket challenge? It just funded an ALS breakthrough. *The Guardian*. Retrieved from www.theguardian.com/society/2016/jul/26/ice-bucket-challenge-als-charity-gene-discovery

6 Ellison, N. B., Steinfield, C., & Lampe, C. (2007). The benefits of Facebook "Friends": Social capital and college students' use of online social network sites. *Journal of Computer-Mediated Communication*, 12(4), 1143–1168. https://doi.org/10.1111/j.1083-6101.2007.00367.x

7 Piwek, L., & Joinson, A. (2016). "What do they snapchat about?" Patterns of use in time-limited instant messaging service. *Computers in Human Behavior*, 54, 358–367. https://doi.org/10.1016/j.chb.2015.08.026

8 Foley, M. (2016, May 24). What is a Snapchat streak? Here's everything you need to know about Snapstreaks. *Bustle*. Retrieved from www.bustle.com/articles/162803-what-is-a-snapchat-streak-heres-everything-you-need-to-know-about-snapstreaks

9 Dunbar, R. I. M. (1992). Neocortex size as a constraint on group size in primates. *Journal of Human Evolution*, 22(6), 469–493. https://doi.org/10.1016/0047-2484(92)90081-J

10 Dunbar, R. I. M. (2016). Do online social media cut through the constraints that limit the size of offline social networks? *Royal Society Open Science*, 3(1), 1–9. https://doi.org/10.1098/rsos.150292

11 Marwick, A. E., & boyd, danah. (2010). I tweet honestly, I tweet passionately: Twitter users, context collapse, and the imagined audience. *New Media & Society*, 13(1), 114–133. https://doi.org/10.1177/1461444810365313

12 Festl, R., & Quandt, T. (2013). Social relations and cyberbullying: The influence of individual and structural attributes on victimization and perpetration via the internet. *Human Communication Research*, 39(1), 101–126. https://doi.org/10.1111/j.1468-2958.2012.01442.x

13 Przybylski, A. K., Murayama, K., Dehaan, C. R., & Gladwell, V. (2013). Motivational, emotional, and behavioral correlates of fear of missing out. *Computers in Human Behavior*, 29(4), 1841–1848. https://doi.org/10.1016/j.chb.2013.02.014

FURTHER READING

Beer, D. (2016). *Metric power*. London: Palgrave Macmillan.

boyd, danah. (2014). *It's complicated: The social lives of networked teens*. New Haven, CT: Yale University Press.

Danziger, K. (1997). *Naming the mind: How psychology found its language*. London: Sage.

De Vos, J. (2013). *Psychologization and the subject of late modernity*. London: Palgrave Macmillan.

Howard, P., & Wooley, S. (eds.) (2018). *Computational propaganda: Political parties, politicians, and political manipulation on social media*. Oxford: Oxford University Press.

Hughes, B. (2018). *Psychology in crisis*. London: Red Globe Press.

Livingstone, S., & Blum-Ross, A. (forthcoming). *Parenting for a digital future*. Oxford: Oxford University Press.

Marwick, A. E. (2013). *Status update: Celebrity, publicity and branding in the social media age*. New Haven, CT: Yale University Press.

Rainie, L., & Wellman, B. (2012). *Networked: The new social operating system*. Cambridge, MA: MIT Press.

Rose, N. (1989). *Governing the soul*. London: Free Association Books.

Suler, J. R. (2015). *Psychology of the digital age: Humans become electric*. Cambridge: Cambridge University Press.

Taylor, C. (1989). *Sources of the self: The making of modern identity*. Cambridge, MA: Harvard University Press.

Vaidhyanathan, S. (2018). *Antisocial media: How Facebook disconnects us and undermines democracy*. Oxford: Oxford University Press.

van Dijck, J. (2013). *The culture of connectivity: A critical history of social media*. Oxford: Oxford University Press.

3

WHEN DO PEOPLE BELIEVE CONSPIRACY THEORIES?

JAN-WILLEM VAN PROOIJEN

"How do you explain the fact that conspiracy theories are on the rise nowadays?" This is a question that I get exceptionally often – from students, from members of an audience after giving a talk, or from journalists who are writing a newspaper article on conspiracy theories. The answer often surprises people: I don't think that conspiracy theories are on the rise. Surely there is some waxing and waning of conspiracy theories throughout the decades. In that respect I am perfectly open to the possibility that in 2016 – with Donald Trump spreading conspiracy theories during the entire US election and the UK voting in favor of a "Brexit" – conspiracy theories have received more attention than in, say, 2006. But I dispute the assertion that there is a stable trend towards more conspiracy theories in the long run. On average, the current population is not more or less conspiratorial than 30, or even 100, years ago. Scientific evidence offers little support for the idea that people have become more conspiratorial over time.

In what I regard as one of the most important, and certainly one of the most labor-intensive, studies on conspiracy theories that has been conducted so far, two political scientists from the University of Miami (helped by a team of trained research assistants) analyzed published letters that US citizens had sent to the Chicago Tribune and the New York Times.[1] The letters spanned a time period of 120 years, ranging from

1890 to 2010. Each year was about equally represented in the sample of letters, and the letters to be analyzed were randomly selected out of all the letters that were published during this period. Of primary interest to the researchers was the extent to which these letters contained conspiracy theories. In the end, these researchers read, and coded for conspiratorial content, a total of 104,803 published letters.

As might be expected, there is variation across the years in the extent to which the letters contain conspiratorial content; furthermore, in different time periods people wrote about different conspiracy theories. But over time, there was no trend upwards in the proportion of letters that contained conspiracy theories. In fact, there were two time periods that seemed to stand out in frequency of conspiratorial content, but both were not in the new millennium. The first time period when there was evidence for increased conspiratorial content was around the year 1900, during the peak of the Second Industrial Revolution. The second time period when there was evidence for increased conspiratorial content was in the late 1940s–early 1950s: at the start of the Cold War. These data clearly speak against assertions that conspiracy theories are on the rise.

Necessarily there are minor imperfections of this study that people could seize on to discredit its importance. For instance, one might reason that the letters that were actually published in these newspapers were selected by an editor and hence were not random. Some editors may have been more likely to publish conspiratorial letters than others. These are unavoidable limitations of a project like this. But we should also be realistic: This is an enormous number of letters, published in two different newspapers, selected by many different editors, over a range of a full 120 years. If there is any merit to the statement that conspiracy theories are on the rise in our modern age, there should be some trace of this visible in these data. For instance, if digital communication technologies make citizens more susceptible to conspiracy theories, the letters should show an increase in conspiratorial content starting somewhere in the early '90s and gradually increasing until the last year of measurement (2010). The data show none of this.

Also other data contradict the idea that people nowadays are more suspicious of power holders than they were about 30 years go. One study looked at the extent to which people trust and are satisfied with politicians in various EU countries over time using yearly data of the Eurobarometer.[2] Particularly the data on satisfaction are of interest, as they range from well before regular citizens had Internet, social media, and smartphones (1974) until a time when these technologies were a normal part of everyday life (2012) (the data on trust are less telling, as these ranged from 1997 to 2012 – although it is worth noting that also in these data no trend emerged suggesting a decline in trust over time). Although admittedly dissatisfaction with politicians is not the same as believing in a political conspiracy theory, one is highly likely to be diagnostic for the other: People are dissatisfied with politicians if they believe that these politicians are conspiring (and vice versa). Again, the results revealed fluctuation in the extent to which citizens were satisfied or dissatisfied with politicians, but there was no trend suggesting a drop in satisfaction levels as time progressed. Furthermore, throughout the years the average satisfaction level that citizens expressed about politicians was quite low. It would thus be a mistake to think that citizens nowadays are less satisfied with politicians than ever before. Back in the 1970s, citizens were also very much dissatisfied with politicians and, apparently, to about an equal extent as nowadays.

All of this may seem counterintuitive. After all, conspiracy theories are everywhere on the Internet and on Social Media, and these modern tools are primary means through which people learn about conspiracy theories or get into contact with other conspiracy theorists. Note that I am not saying that modern information technologies have no impact. But there is a difference between speed of dissemination and the proportion of citizens who believe conspiracy theories. My prediction would be that these modern communication technologies increase the speed through which people learn about conspiracy theories but do not increase the proportion of citizens who believe them. In a time when citizens did not have Internet or social media at their disposal, conspiracy theories were likely to spread through different, slower communication channels (e.g., word of mouth), but major conspiracy theories would spread nevertheless and ultimately reach most people anyway.

Certainly conspiracy theories spread fast nowadays. On 2 December 2015 the San Bernardino (California) shootings took place in the late morning. A married couple killed 14 people and injured another 22 with semi-automatic rifles. After the shooting, a manhunt ensued which lasted for about four hours, after which both perpetrators were killed. As the event unfolded it was evening in Amsterdam, where I was watching live coverage of this event on TV together with my wife. About two hours after the start of the shooting (and hence, two hours *before* the perpetrators were killed) I could not resist the temptation and Googled something like "San Bernardino conspiracy". Instantly various conspiracy theories came up suggesting that the shooting was a false-flag operation. We could read conspiracy theories about this terrorist attack while it was still unfolding! Without modern communication technology, however, these conspiracy theories may have reached us too, eventually – or alternatively, in Amsterdam we might not have heard about the San Bernardino shooting in the first place, and we would instead have focused more on local distressing events (leading to local conspiracy theories). Modern information technologies play a role in conspiracy theories, but when we seek answers to the question why people believe or disbelieve them, these technologies are only a piece in a much bigger puzzle.

Instead of seeking an explanation in "zeitgeist" or technology, a better and more comprehensive explanation for conspiracy beliefs can be found in psychology. I propose that conspiracy theories are rooted in a subjective psychological state that has been inherent to the human condition since the start of humanity: Conspiracy theories are a natural reaction to social situations that elicit feelings of fear and uncertainty. Specifically, the more strongly people experience such aversive emotions, the more likely it is that they assign blame for distressing events to different groups. As a consequence, we can expect conspiracy theories particularly in the wake of distressing societal events.

CONSPIRACY THEORIES AND SOCIETAL CRISIS SITUATIONS

People regularly are confronted with societal crisis situations – rapid changes in society that could potentially threaten their well-being, their way of life, or even their existence. Examples of such crisis situations are terrorist attacks, natural disasters, wars, revolutions, economic and financial crises, disease epidemics, and the like. Such crisis situations almost invariably lead to conspiracy theories. Two key examples of sudden, unexpected crises in modern history that inspired widespread conspiracy theories are the 9/11 terrorist strikes and the assassination of John F. Kennedy. Both were events that shocked society, that installed strong feelings of fear and uncertainty in people, and that gave people the feeling that the world would never be the same again. Many people have "flashbulb memories" about these events, as they still vividly recall what they were doing when they first heard the news. Both events also initiated conspiracy theories that are still being endorsed today by large groups of citizens and that many people by now have internalized as historical "facts".

The two spikes that emerged in conspiratorial content within the letters sent to the *New York Times* and *Chicago Tribune* can also be regarded as crisis situations that formed the basis of feelings of uncertainty and fear. The first spike with increased conspiracy beliefs was during the Second Industrial Revolution. During this time period major companies started to emerge, and power structures within society changed dramatically. It was a time of rapid technological progress, quick development of new infrastructure, and the efficient mass-production of a wide range of goods. Although life conditions improved for many citizens, regular laborers who were working in factories had reason for concern: There was a continuous threat of unemployment, as many jobs became obsolete after being replaced by machines. It is quite likely that these workers – who constituted a large portion of the population – experienced substantial uncertainty about their future, producing a range of conspiracy theories. The second spike with increased conspiracy beliefs was at the start of the Cold War. Shortly after the Second World War many citizens feared the prospect of a new major war, and the threat of communism was looming. As a consequence, many citizens were wary of the possibility that specific people, institutions, or groups were somehow connected to communism. This "McCarthyism" – named after senator Joseph McCarthy who was a significant figure in fueling fear of communism – was hence characterized by many (often unfounded) allegations of communist conspiracies within society. These communist conspiracy theories caused reputation damage, unemployment, and sometimes even imprisonment of people who were accused of communist sympathies.

But we do not need to restrict ourselves to the past century in order to find a connection between crisis situations and conspiracy theories. Also in the Middle Ages, examples abound of crisis situations that initiated widespread belief in conspiracy theories. Medical science was not as advanced as our current generation is used to, and it was common for young children to die of a range of dangerous diseases that nowadays are easily prevented with vaccines. Furthermore, there was no understanding of viruses or bacteria (or the importance of personal hygiene for that matter), and antibiotics were yet to be discovered. As a consequence, disease epidemics were frequent and would kill many people, but people were unable to fully understand how these diseases originated. People therefore often blamed these epidemics on people or groups in society, and such scapegoating regularly took the form of conspiracy theories. One common belief was that many young women were actually witches who conspired with the Devil to impose harm on the population such as epidemics or failed harvests. As a result of these beliefs – which are both superstitious and conspiratorial – many innocent women were burnt alive. Also the Jewish community was a frequent target of conspiracy theories suggesting that they had a causal role in crisis situations such as disease epidemics or setbacks during the Crusades, stimulating widespread persecution of Jews in Medieval Europe.[3]

These are just examples of a more general principle: In challenging times that elicit fear and uncertainty among large groups of people, conspiracy theories flourish. People start blaming people or groups that they felt uncomfortable about to begin with and come up with theories that explain the harm they experience through a malevolent conspiracy. As a result, conspiracy theories will increase in the population once there is widespread concern about a high-profile terrorist attack, a natural disaster, an economic or financial crisis, a war, a revolution, and so on. Events that pose no direct threat to peoples' own lives also can stimulate conspiracy theories, as long as it captures the attention of a large audience and causes feelings of distress among many citizens (e.g., the unexpected death of a celebrity).

In fact, even imaginary crisis situations can cause conspiracy beliefs. A case in point is the conspiracy theory that the 1969 moon landings were filmed in a TV studio. One might reason that these conspiracy theories were not a reaction to an "objective" crisis situation – it was a reaction to a positive event where humanity and science reached a new level of accomplishment. But someone who believes that the government continuously and willfully deceives the nation subjectively experiences the nation as being in crisis. Put differently, many people hold general conspiratorial beliefs about the government, and these beliefs are distressing in and of themselves, which causes further conspiracy theorizing. This is a general insight that I will return to in other chapters: Belief in one conspiracy theory stimulates belief in other conspiracy theories. In this case, citizens who hold conspiracy theories about the government are likely to approach any action of that government – including a monument to scientific accomplishment like the moon landings – with skepticism, and with additional conspiracy theories.

THE ROLE OF FEAR AND UNCERTAINTY

In order to understand why feelings of uncertainty and fear are associated with conspiracy theories, we need to establish how people cope with these negative emotions. The most common response to fear and uncertainty is to become vigilant: People start paying close attention to their environment, they start to ruminate, and they try to establish the causes of their negative feelings. Fear and uncertainty thus lead people to try to make sense of their physical and social environment.[4] Such increased sense making is an automatic response that in all likelihood is rooted in an instinct for self-preservation. Feelings of fear and uncertainty signal that there are imminent threats in the environment. Paying close attention to this environment therefore increases the chances of the organism to effectively cope with these threats and survive.

As part of this self-preservation instinct, evolutionary psychologists have noted that people tend to be risk-averse in the face of uncertain and possibly threatening situations.[5] Imagine seeing a long object in the grass, and it is unclear whether the object is a stick or a snake. In such cases, it is a natural response for people to be cautious and assume the object to be a snake. Mistakes do not have equal consequences in this situation: Someone who picks up the object assuming it to be a stick may die if it turns out to be a venomous snake. But for someone who assumes the object to be a snake and hence acts cautiously, it does not matter whether that judgment is correct or not. If one is mistaken and the snake is in fact a stick, one may take an unnecessary detour, but for the rest no real harm is done.

Feelings of uncertainty lead people to make sense of the situation that they find themselves in, and during this mental sense making it is natural for them to assume the worst. This also pertains to how people perceive others. One common finding in psychology is the "myth of self-interest". Just for clarification, this term does not mean that self-interest is a myth; of course people can be selfish from time to time. Instead, this term means that people *overestimate* the extent to which the behavior of *others* is driven by self-interest. People can be selfish sometimes, but they can also be genuinely altruistic and caring – but when trying to explain the behavior of others, people more often assume selfishness and less often assume truly benevolent motivations than is actually justified. (When Mark Zuckerberg decided to donate 99% of his Facebook shares to charity, I was astonished to read one blog after the other of people who believed him to do this out of self-interest.)

Interestingly, this myth of self-interest increases when people feel uncertain. In an experiment, participants were informed that a second participant would allocate valuable recourses between the two of them. To a varying extent, however, participants experienced uncertainty in the form of lacking information: They were not fully informed about how the allocator distributed the resources. Results showed that this informational uncertainty led participants to over-estimate the valuable resources that the allocators had given to them-selves and to underestimate the valuable resources that the allocators had given to the participants. People expected the allocators to be more selfish than they actually were, and this effect increased to the extent that people had less information about the distributions. As the authors conclude, when people lack information they "fill in the blanks" with assumptions of selfishness.[6]

This myth of self-interest is about how negatively people view other individuals, but through a similar process, feelings of fear and uncertainty also influence how negatively people view other groups in society. When making sense of the societal and political events that people encounter in their daily life, people have a tendency to assume the worst of groups that are powerful (and that could hence cause real harm), that they perceive as "different", and that they feel uncomfort-able with – such as governmental institutions, major companies, or distrusted minority groups. As a result, people come up with con-spiracy theories about the malpractice of these groups, which answers many unresolved questions that people have about the societal events that they try to comprehend. Feelings of uncertainty and fear put people in a suspicious, information-seeking state-of-mind, leading them to perceive malevolent conspiracies as responsible for a range of societal events.

Much psychological research has examined the relationship between fearful, uncertain feelings and people's tendency to believe conspiracy theories. One study was conducted in the last three months of 1999. During those months, many citizens around the world feared a major shutdown of computer systems due to the "millennium bug". This was a major issue at the time. The possibility of a millennium bug received continuous news coverage, and people feared major fallout of for instance power plants, banking systems, water supplies, and the like. If these fears had been justified and the millennium bug had become a reality, it would have had serious consequences for the economy, health care, and many other domains that directly influence the life and well-being of citizens: Anything that was run by computers would shut down. (In the end, the year 2000 started without unusual problems.) Against this background, over 1,200 US citizens responded to a questionnaire that not only asked how afraid they were for the millennium bug but also to what extent they believed in a range of common conspiracy theories. As it turned out, people who feared the millennium bug by the end of 1999 were also more likely to believe that President Kennedy was killed by a conspiracy; that the Air Force was hiding evidence that the US has been visited by UFOs; that the US government deliberately had put drugs in inner city communities; and that the Japanese were conspiring to destroy the US economy. Fear for the millennium bug was associated with belief in a range of conspiracy theories, including theories that are conceptually unconnected with the millennium bug.[7]

While these findings support the idea that feelings of fear are related with belief in conspiracy theories, they do not establish causality: We do not know whether fear of the millennium bug increased conspiracy beliefs or, instead, people who happened to believe these conspiracy theories were more likely to fear the millennium bug. In order to test for the causal order that fear and uncertainty lead to conspiracy theories, it is necessary to conduct a psychological experiment in which part of the research participants experience these distressing feelings and part of the research participants do not – and then examine whether belief in conspiracy theories is stronger among the distressed participants. Various studies tried to install these distressing feelings in participants by reminding them of situations in which they experienced a lack of control. Specifically, people have a need to feel that they are in control of whatever they do, ranging from simple movements to more complex actions such as driving a car. If people experience a lack of control they feel helpless and therefore start feeling uncertain. In a typical experiment, some of the research participants are asked to write down a specific incident in their lives where they had no control over the situation; other research participants are asked to write down a specific incident in their lives where they were in full control of the situation. After that, they are asked how plausible they find certain conspiracy theories.

Various researchers have conducted experiments along these lines, and these studies typically show that people believe in conspiracy theories more strongly when they feel distressed (e.g., because they were reminded of a situation where they lacked control) than when they do not feel distressed (e.g., because they were reminded of a situation where they had control).[8] Together with psychologist Michele Acker and a group of research assistants, we also conducted such an experiment in Amsterdam. The experiment took place against the background of the construction of a new and controversial metro line that would connect the northern and southern part of the city. Although such a metro line is likely to have many benefits once completed, it encountered severe objections among Amsterdam residents, as it would imply major construction works for years, right through the historical center. In fact, a majority of residents had voted against this project in a referendum, but the city council moved forward with it anyway. Furthermore, the construction itself ran into many problems, including being overbudget and behind schedule. Public hostility against this project reached its peak in 2009, when the construction caused unforeseen problems that posed direct harm to city residents: The underground construction had damaged the foundations of several old houses, which then had to be evacuated, as the houses literally were sinking into the ground.

When the "sinking houses" made continuous news headlines, our team of research assistants went to university cafeterias in

Amsterdam with short questionnaires and asked residents to participate in a short study in exchange for a candy bar. Participants were asked to describe either a situation from their lives where they lacked control or one where they had full control. A third group of participants were asked to describe a neutral situation from their lives, unrelated to feelings of fear or uncertainty. Then we asked participants about their conspiracy theories of the North-South Metro line: For instance, participants indicated whether they believed that members of the city council were bribed by the construction companies, whether they deliberately withheld information about the project from the public to avoid hampering its construction, and so on. In keeping with many other findings, results revealed that participants who felt fearful and uncertain (after describing a situation where they lacked control) believed these conspiracy theories more strongly than participants who felt confident (after describing a situation where they had control).[9]

In sum, feelings of fear and uncertainty fuel belief in conspiracy theories. Yet there are two complications to these effects that deserve to be noted. A first complication is that these aversive emotions do not lead to conspiracy theories among everyone and in every circumstance: Sometimes fear and uncertainty can actually *increase* support for authorities. So far we have discussed the conspiracy theories that emerged after 9/11, but we should also recognize the opposite: In the months directly after 9/11, George W. Bush was among the most positively endorsed presidents in history in terms of public approval ratings. Apparently, 9/11 not only elicited widespread conspiracy theories about the Bush administration; it also elicited massive support for the Bush administration. How can we reconcile this discrepancy with the present arguments?

The key here is that fear and uncertainty lead to conspiracy theories, but only if these theories involve powerful groups or institutions that people distrusted to begin with. Fear and uncertainty may actually increase support for powerful groups or institutions that people do trust. One study investigated whether or not the perception of leaders being moral or immoral influences belief in conspiracy theories. Naturally, people believe conspiracy theories more strongly about leaders that they find immoral than about leaders that they find moral. When people experience uncertainty, however, these effects of morality on belief in conspiracy theories become more impactful. Put differently, uncertainty makes people endorse conspiracy theories more strongly for leaders that they find immoral but less strongly for leaders that they find moral.[10] Fear and uncertainty hence do not lead to indiscriminate conspiracy theorizing; they lead people to place blame on authorities, institutions, or groups that they felt uncomfortable with from the start.

The second complication is that, often, also the "official" explanation of a crisis event entails a conspiracy. The official reading of the 9/11 strikes is that there was a conspiracy of 19 Al Qaeda suicide terrorists. Why did many citizens disbelieve this official reading and instead perceived a different conspiracy of a malevolent government performing a false-flag operation? Two interrelated issues may answer this question. First, as noted previously, when people experience fear and uncertainty, it is their natural response to be cautious and assume the worst possible explanation. In that sense, believing that 9/11 was a governmental conspiracy (and not an Al Qaeda conspiracy) is a risk-averse response: It is a lot more disturbing, frightening, and dangerous to assume that one's own government would be behind a major terrorist act, as compared to a known foreign terrorist group that is being closely monitored by secret service agencies. Second, and relatedly, a governmental conspiracy is a more grandiose explanation for 9/11 than an Al Qaeda terrorist cell: It would for instance mean that more people were involved, the level of deception would be bigger, and the scheme that was carried out would be more ingenious, and in general a government has more power than a terrorist cell. The 9/11 terrorist strikes constituted a major event in modern history, and a governmental conspiracy would be a major explanation for it. The tendency to believe a grandiose conspiracy theory may be influenced by a basic heuristic of the human mind called the proportionality bias: People have a tendency to assume that a big consequence must have had a big cause.

BIG CONSEQUENCES, BIG CAUSES?

A president is a human being, and is therefore fragile enough to die from accidents or sudden illnesses. It is perfectly possible for an otherwise healthy president to die from a tiny flu virus, just like everyone else. Now, imagine for a moment that this would actually happen to a sitting US president or a UK prime minister. Would many citizens believe that this event indeed was caused by a simple virus, or would they believe a conspiracy theory? Although certainly the opinions would differ among the public, and a lot would depend upon specific details of the case, in general I am quite confident that many citizens would come up with major conspiracy theories asserting that the president was murdered (or was kidnapped, or staged his/her own death). The explanation of an event as big as the death of a president through a cause as small as a flu virus is just hard to swallow for many people: It cannot possibly be this simple, there must be more to such an impactful, world-changing event than that. This is the essence of the proportionality bias: the assumption that a big consequence must have had a big cause.

Naturally, the unexpected death of a president would elicit strong feelings of fear and uncertainty among the population. But the proportionality bias is also broader than regulating these aversive feelings: It is a simple mental heuristic that can be seen across judgment domains, also in areas unrelated to conspiracy theories that do not elicit fear and uncertainty. Imagine two comparable students that both experience a computer crash right before having to hand in an important paper. For the first student, the consequences are disastrous: The professor fails the student for the class and does not grant an extension for the paper; this leads the student to not graduate in time and to therefore lose an attractive job offer. For the second student, the consequences are relatively small: The professor allows the student an extension to hand in the paper. As a result the student does graduate in time and can start with the attractive job. What may have caused the computer crash for the first and second student?

In a research study, half of the participants read a hypothetical scenario of the first student, and the other half read a scenario of the second student. They then selected what they thought was the most likely cause of the crash: a widespread computer virus (big cause) or a malfunctioning computer cooling fan (small cause). Research participants massively recognized a widespread computer virus as a bigger computer problem than a malfunctioning fan. But more importantly, when the consequences were big for the student, research participants were more likely to believe that the computer crash had a big cause – that is, a computer virus. These findings are unlikely to be explained by fear and uncertainty: After all, these were hypothetical scenarios of an unknown student. Instead, the proportionality bias was at work here: Participants assumed a big cause for a big consequence – in this case, a computer virus if the crash caused the student to fail his studies.[11]

The proportionality bias similarly has been shown to influence people's tendency to believe conspiracy theories. Imagine that a president of a small country gets assassinated. In one case, this assassination instigates an unforeseen chain of events ultimately leading to a war. In the other case, the assassination may still be tragic, but does not lead to a war. Put differently, the assassination has a big consequence (a war) or not. Who assassinated the president – was it a lone gunman, or was it a governmental conspiracy? A study revealed that participants considered a conspiracy more likely if the assassination led to a war than if it did not lead to a war. Again, people assumed a big cause for a big consequence, which in this case fueled a conspiracy theory. Various other studies suggest a similar principle: The more impactful and harmful a societal event is (including hypothetical ones), the more likely it is that people come up with a conspiracy theory to explain it.

Besides fear and uncertainty, the proportionality bias constitutes an additional explanation for the observation that we particularly can expect conspiracy theories in the wake of impactful, harmful societal events. Note that both the emotional explanation (fear and uncertainty) as well as the cognitive explanation (the proportionality bias) are rooted in people's desire to understand and make sense of the harmful events that they perceive in society. Sense making thus is essential in the psychology of conspiracy theories. In the following chapter, I will more precisely uncover the mental processes that are at work when people make sense of societal events – and how these may lead to conspiracy theories.

NOTES

1 Uscinksi & Parent, 2014
2 Andeweg, 2014
3 Pipes, 1997
4 Park, 2010
5 Neuberg, Kenrick, & Schaller, 2011
6 Vuolevi & Van Lange, 2010
7 Van Prooijen & Acker, 2015
8 Sullivan et al., 2010; Van Harreveld et al., 2014; Whitson & Galinsky, 2008
9 Van Prooijen & Acker, 2015
10 Van Prooijen & Jostmann, 2013
11 Leboeuf & Norton, 2012

REFERENCES

Andeweg, R. B. (2014). A growing confidence gap in politics? Data versus discourse. In J.-W. van Prooijen & P. A. M. van Lange (Eds.), *Power, politics, and paranoia: Why people are suspicious of their leaders* (pp. 176–198). Cambridge, UK: Cambridge University Press.

LeBoeuf, R. A., & Norton, M. I. (2012). Consequence-cause matching: Looking to the consequences of events to infer their causes. *Journal of Consumer Research, 39*, 128–141.

Neuberg, S. L., Kenrick, D. T., & Schaller, M. (2011). Human threat management systems: Self-protection and disease avoidance. *Neuroscience and Biobehavioral Reviews, 35*, 1042–1051.

Park, C. L. (2010). Making sense of the meaning literature: An integrative review of meaning making and its effects on adjustment to stressful life events. *Psychological Bulletin, 136*, 257–301.

Pipes, D. (1997). *Conspiracy: How the paranoid style flourishes and where it comes from.* New York, NY: Simon & Schuster.

Sullivan, D., Landau, M. J., & Rothschild, Z. K. (2010). An existential function of enemyship: Evidence that people attribute influence to personal and political enemies to compensate for threats to control. *Journal of Personality and Social Psychology, 98,* 434–449.

Uscinski, J. E., & Parent, J. M. (2014). *American conspiracy theories.* New York, NY: Oxford University Press.

Van Harreveld, F., Rutjens, B. T., Schneider, I. K., Nohlen, H. U., & Keskinis, K. (2014). In doubt and disorderly: Ambivalence promotes compensatory perceptions of order. *Journal of Experimental Psychology: General, 143,* 1666–1676.

Van Prooijen, J.-W., & Acker, M. (2015). The influence of control on belief in conspiracy theories: Conceptual and applied extensions. *Applied Cognitive Psychology, 29,* 753–761.

Van Prooijen, J.-W., & Jostmann, N. B. (2013). Belief in conspiracy theories: The influence of uncertainty and perceived morality. *European Journal of Social Psychology, 43,* 109–115.

Vuolevi, J. H. K., & Van Lange, P. A. M. (2010). Beyond the information given: The power of a belief in self-interest. *European Journal of Social Psychology, 40,* 26–34.

Whitson, J. A., & Galinsky, A. D. (2008). Lacking control increases illusory pattern perception. *Science, 322,* 115–117.

FURTHER READING

Books about conspiracy theories

- For an interesting popular science book about conspiracy theories, read *Suspicious minds: Why we believe conspiracy theories* by Rob Brotheron (2015; New York, NY: Bloomsbury Sigma).
- For a US political science perspective, read *American conspiracy theories* by Joseph E. Uscinski and Joseph M. Parent (2014; New York, NY: Oxford University Press). This book also contains the study that analyzes more than 100,000 letters over a time period of 120 years, described in Chapter 2 .
- For a historical perspective on conspiracy theories, read *Conspiracy: How the paranoid style fl ourishes and where it comes from* by Daniel Pipes (1997; New York, NY: Simon & Schuster).
- Also of interest is the political-historical approach of *Political paranoia: The psychopolitics of hatred* by Robert S. Robins and Jerrold M. Post (1997; New Haven, CT: Yale University Press).
- For a volume on conspiracy theories in which multiple authors offer their view, read *The psychology of conspiracy* edited by Michal Bilewicz, Aleksandra Cichocka, and Wiktor Soral (2015; Oxon, UK: Routledge).
- For a volume in which various authors address not only conspiracy theories but also the question whether power really does corrupt, read *Power, politics, and paranoia: Why people are suspicious of their leaders* edited by Jan-Willem van Prooijen and Paul A. M. van Lange (2014; Cambridge, UK: Cambridge University Press).

Books about belief in general

- For an excellent popular science book about the ideas in Chapter 3 on the architecture of beliefs, read *The believing brain: From ghosts and*

gods to politics and conspiracies – How we construct beliefs and reinforce them as truths by Michael Shermer (2011; New York, NY: Henry Holt).
- Another good popular science book on the psychology of belief is " *The belief instinct: The psychology of souls, destiny, and the meaning of life* " by Jesse Bering (2011; New York, NY: W.W. Norton & Co).

Books about populism/extremism and conspiracy theories

- For a good introduction to populism, read *What is populism?* by Jan-Werner Müller (2016; Philadelphia, PA: University of Pennsylvania Press). The book also addresses the role of conspiracy theories in populist movements.
- For the qualitative study on extremist fringe groups and conspiracy theories, read *The power of unreason: Conspiracy theories, extremism and counterterrorism* by Jamie Bartlett, J. and Carl Miller (2010; London, UK: Demos).

Books about belief versus reality

- Do some of the pseudo-scientifi c "9/11 for truth" conspiracy theories appear plausible to you? Then defi nitely read *Debunking 9/11 myths: Why conspiracy theories can't stand up to the facts* by David Dunbar and Brad Reagan (2011; New York, NY: Hearst Books). In it, you will learn what scientists and witnesses actually have to say about the conspiracy theories associated with this event.
- Do you feel that there may be a grain of truth in some paranormal phenomena? Please learn about the scientifi c evidence in *Paranormality: The science of the supernatural* by Richard Wiseman (2011; London, UK: Pan Books).

Other

- Watch how a blacksmith refutes the 9/11 "melted steel" conspiracy theory described in Chapter 6: www.youtube.com/watch?v= FzF1KySHmUA
- See the TV interview in which Prince talks about chemtrails, described in Chapter 1: http://youtu.be/3zEiAQdyAGk
- Read an interview with the author, about the psychology of conspiracy theories: www.vox.com/science-and-health/2017/4/25/15408610/conspiracy-theories-psychologist-explained

4 The dynamics of groups online

Olivia Hurley

CHAPTER OVERVIEW

This chapter outlines how online groups form and regulate themselves. It examines the dynamics of online groups compared to their offline counterparts, focusing on why online group membership is an attractive option for many people, especially in today's digital age. Specifically, the chapter addresses topics such as how roles, norms and group identity are expressed in online groups. Other recent research areas, such as the impact of an over-reliance on online social networks on individuals' mental well-being, and the phenomenon of groupthink related to online groups, are also presented.

KEY TERMS

Collective identity describes how people are similar to each other, when the psychological connection between the individual self and the social group the individual is a member of is considered. **Groupthink** refers to 'the tendency for cohesive groups to become so concerned about group consolidation that they fail to critically and realistically evaluate their decisions and antecedent assumptions' (Park, 1990, p. 229). **Group norms** are the rules individuals are expected to obey as members of a particular group, while **group roles** are the parts that individuals play within a group, or the positions they fill within a group, both formal and informal. **Social loafing** describes the reduction in effort exerted by some individuals when performing a task as part of a group, compared to completing the task alone.

INTRODUCTION

This chapter outlines how online groups form and regulate themselves. Some key questions one might be interested in posing when considering this topic of groups online could include: What is the psychological impact of being a member of an online group, such as a Facebook group, a Twitter group, or being a LinkedIn member, compared with being a member of an offline group – for example, in a physical work setting or a sports club setting? Are people more likely to join groups online than they would be to join a similar group offline? Are online groups more or less homogeneous – that is, do individuals in online groups share more common characteristics with other group members, when compared to similar offline groups? Are shy people really 'bolder' or 'braver' online? In order to answer such questions, one must first understand what a group is, how it is formed and why such groups form.

What is a group? How and why do groups form?

A group is any collection of people in a particular location or setting. Most people are considered members of many groups during their lifetime, such as their class group, their work group, or, more common in today's digital age, a member of an online group, such as an online social networking group (Kirwan & Power, 2014). The question of how and why groups form has been investigated for decades, perhaps most frequently by social psychologists, such as Maslow (1943), who, in his paper 'The theory of human motivation', described how human beings have 'needs', which are prioritised, with physical needs and safety needs positioned at the bottom levels of a hypothetical pyramid that he had suggested, followed by love and belonging needs. These love and belonging needs refer to the human 'need' to be cared for, to form social bonds, and to seek out contact with other human beings. Such needs are considered fundamental to what it means to be human. So, human beings are considered social creatures with a need to 'belong', to be accepted by their peers, to be valued, yet unique individuals, with common goals and interests compared to other group members (Baumeister & Leary, 1995). This social need to 'belong' appears to be a strong motivating factor for why many people join groups, including groups in the online world (Chiu *et al.*, 2008). However, online group membership is determined by more than just social factors. It is also determined by users' access to the necessary technology to enable them to join and interact in such groups, and their usability skills for such technology (Daneback *et al.*, 2012). So, having addressed some of the issues surrounding what groups are, and what motivates individuals to join groups, the reasons why individuals join online groups specifically, and group behaviours online will now be discussed.

Why do individuals join online groups?

According to researchers such as Code and Zaparyniuk (2009), and Kirwan and Power (2014), some of most common reasons for joining online groups include, first, the *need to alleviate loneliness* (whether that is temporary, such as moving to a new city, or chronic, such as being housebound for long periods of time due to ill health, for example), and second, the attraction of the *relative anonymity* that such online groups provide, which may be especially appealing for shy individuals, such as those struggling with social anxiety disorders (Kirwan & Power, 2014), or those who wish to control the *amount and type of self-disclosures* they provide to other members of their social groups. People with social anxiety disorders, for example, who find it difficult to interact in groups in everyday real life, may find the online community a more attractive option for them in which to interact with others because they may feel safer, and more at ease expressing themselves online as they are not required to be physically present for such interactions to take place. Similarly, individuals' anxieties regarding the reactions of others in their offline world, to their '*different*' or '*special*' *interests*, could result in such individuals being, or feeling, ostracised and isolated from their offline, real world, peer groups, thus accounting perhaps for their, and a third motivation, to seek out like-minded individuals online to converse with instead (Bargh & McKenna, 2004; Kirwan & Power, 2014; Walther, 2007).

A fourth attraction to joining online groups is their ability to allow individuals to *communicate remotely* with other members of a group they share perhaps a common predicament or problem with, or when time to meet in person is not possible due to time constraints, work/family commitments, or location difficulties – i.e. living in a remote place with little public transport services. There is no need to be in the same location or face to face with group members in order to communicate online in such situations. However, many visual cues – for example, body language – are often lost in such online interactions (i.e. those that are type-based communications, via email or message boards). Such non-verbal cues in face-to-face exchanges are considered to add to the richness of the discourse taking place between the group members (Riva, 2002). The loss of visual contact between online group members can mean a loss of understanding of the discourse, in its meaning and context, by individuals who only have written words, and perhaps emoticons, on which to base their interpretations of what is being communicated. However, such typed responses also afford group members the luxury of re-reading their responses before sending them on to other group members, meaning that such responses may be 'toned down' or rephrased in a way that is not truly reflective of what would be said if the group members were engaged in a face to face exchange (Murgado-Armenteros *et al.*, 2012).

Despite the above cited limitation, of typed online group interactions losing their non-verbal cues, such online social communities continue to grow in number and popularity (Kuss & Griffiths, 2011; Facebook, 2012; Van Belleghem *et al.*, 2012). Indeed, the growth of such online communities has resulted in researchers debating the previously held views of how social and psychological dynamics contribute to human relationships, communication and community formation. For example, some early research supported the view that the relative anonymity of Internet communication encourages self-expression and facilitates the formation of relationships outside of what might be considered 'normal' socially mediated communication (Wallace, 1999).

A fifth attraction of online group membership is that the Internet offers a way for individuals to *present a 'version' of themselves* to their group. Identities online are, therefore, sometimes described as 'fluid' or dynamic in nature – that is, they are subject to change, depending on the demands of the online group membership. Indeed, Code and Zaparyniuk (2009) described how individuals often join online groups because this affords them the capacity to experiment and develop their identities in their online groups. Such 'impression management' continues to be extensively researched by cyberpsychologists (Kirwan & Power, 2014).

A sixth attraction of online group membership is perhaps the possibility of forming *multinational groups* as again, cited above, physical contact is not needed to form such online relationships. This ability to communicate with individuals from other countries and cultures opens up a world of interesting exchanges between online group members. However, it is often the case that group members are less spontaneous and more guarded in what they communicate in such multicultural group settings online, as there is perhaps greater uncertainty about the way an exchange in such an environment might be interpreted (Murgado-Armenteros *et al.*, 2012).

The online environment also removes environmental variables, such as room temperature, seating types and arrangements, noise levels – that is, the physical personal space, from the interaction, which may be a favourable feature of online group interactions for individuals who like to control such variables as much as possible. The offline world often places great emphasis on the physical appearance of individuals also, which is removed from interactions in many online settings. This can result in individuals forming bonds with other individuals they share common views and goals with, rather than being related to physical attractiveness, for example. Such relationships may then have greater opportunities to grow in the online world, which could greatly benefit the social bonds of the individuals concerned. Indeed, some early research by Parks and Floyd (1995) reported that people felt the personal relationships they formed via the Internet were close, meaningful and rewarding. This view was supported by McKenna *et al.* (2002) in their two-year longitudinal study of randomly selected Internet newsgroup participants. McKenna *et al.* reported that 84 per cent of their participants claimed that their Internet relationships were as important and 'real' to them as were their non-Internet relationships.

OVER-RELIANCE ON ONLINE GROUP MEMBERSHIP

There are, however, implications for group members who display an over-reliance on their online social groups, such as their 'friends' on social media websites like Facebook, or their 'followers' on Twitter, for example. Melville (2010) reported that individuals may suffer symptoms of depression if they feel rejected by their online 'friends'. Such individuals then risked alienating themselves from their online groups, in a similar fashion to that which may occur with members of groups in their offline world. Also, Kalpidou *et al.* (2011) reported the longer such individuals spend with their online groups in the online world, the lower their self-esteem levels appeared to become offline. However, Kim *et al.* (2009) reported that individuals who scored low on their ability to function in offline social settings declared the beneficial use of online social groups in meeting their unfulfilled social offline group needs. These group members perceived their online groups existed in a 'safer' environment for them. Kim *et al.* did also comment, however, that the difficulties individuals reported having in their offline social interactions, and how they felt about them, were not enhanced, or solved, by participating in online social groups. Therefore, reliance on the online world for social support may result in individuals becoming more socially withdrawn from the offline world, thus facilitating their social anxiety to a greater degree.

Some researchers have specifically tested the psychological impact of denying individuals time to interact on their social networking websites. For example, in their study, Sheldon *et al.* (2011) denied students access to their Facebook accounts for a 48-hour period. These students actually displayed lower levels of aggression and procrastination, while also reporting greater levels of life-satisfaction, for the period they were denied access to their Facebook accounts. They did, however, display a rebound effect in their extended use of Facebook following their 48-hour period of absence from their sites in order, it would appear, to 'make up' for their reported feelings of being 'disconnected' from this online world during the 48-hour period of abstinence imposed during the study.

Gentzler *et al.* (2011) also reported that group members who spent more time interacting with their parents through social media groups displayed higher levels of loneliness and anxious attachment with their parents compared to those who interacted more with their parents in the offline world. The individuals who reported spending more time with their parents in an offline environment stated that their relationships with their parents were more intimate, supportive and satisfying for them, compared to the individuals who interacted more with their parents online.

As previously cited, the Internet and online social networks may provide socially shy individuals with a comfortable environment in which to communicate with others, while avoiding face-to-face interactions (Ebeling-Witte *et al.*, 2007). However, is it true that such individuals are more confident and less self-conscious online? Brunet and Schmidt (2008) attempted to answer this question. They reported that the behaviour and confidence exhibited by shy individuals, who reported being more self-conscious in social settings, was context dependent when they communicated online. For example, when there was a webcam operating, the self-conscious individuals provided less self-disclosure information compared to their less shy counterparts.

To conclude this section, perhaps online groups can provide a peer-supportive forum and a positive environment in which to interact, for some group members, such as those who are shy or self-conscious, or who have special interests. However, some online groups can also be a negative source of social support, especially if they result in feelings of 'disconnectedness', or if they lead to anxious attachments to significant others, such as family and friends in the real world. They can also be damaging, if their online groups encourage, and foster, negative health-related behaviours, such as disordered eating (Tierney, 2006). Such groups can also have a contagion-like effect on vulnerable group members (Lewis & Arbuthnott, 2012).

Having addressed some of the reasons why individuals are motivated to join online groups, and some key advantages and disadvantages of such online group memberships for individuals, the issues of how people behave in groups online, compared to offline, and how such online groups maintain their membership numbers will now be discussed, considering issues such as group identity, roles, norms and social loafing in online groups.

HOW DO PEOPLE BEHAVE IN ONLINE GROUPS?

So, how does group behaviour online differ from group behaviour offline, if indeed any differences do exist? In order to answer such a question, the term 'group dynamics' should first be explained. According to Moran (2012), group dynamics is a term used to describe the way individuals act in groups, the factors thought to influence group behaviour and the processes thought to change group behaviour. But first, what constitutes examples of online groups? In the online world, environments which constitute groups include social networks, such as Facebook, Twitter and Instagram, chat-rooms, email lists, discussion boards, bulletin boards, news and discussion groups, list servers, as well as Massively Multiple Online Role Playing Games (MMORPG; such large groups will be discussed in detail in Chapter 19). The main objective of such online groups is to provide members with a common cyberspace in which to share their experiences, to seek advice, and to communicate with others (Castelnuovo et al., 2003). There are many similarities between such online groups and their offline equivalents (e.g. clubs, societies, gym groups, political groups), such as the need of members for social connections and social support, as outlined earlier in this chapter. However, there are also some key differences between such groups online, compared to similar offline groups (Howard, 2014). So, do online groups serve a different purpose in a person's life, compared to their offline groups? Do individuals fulfil different roles in online groups, when compared to their offline roles in their real-world lives? According to Chmiel et al. (2011), Internet communication patterns do appear to differ when compared to those displayed in traditional, face-to-face settings. Therefore, the influence of cohesion, roles and norms on online group functioning, the types of leadership structures that exist online, and some of the negative features of online group behaviour, such as groupthink and social loafing, will now be discussed.

Online group cohesion

Similar to the concept of team cohesion in sporting and work-related environments (Moran, 2012), group survival in the online world relies on groups sharing some form of task and social cohesion. This means that a group must help an individual to fulfil some objectives or goals (i.e. tasks), while also meeting some interpersonal (or social) needs of the individual, if that individual is to remain a member of the group. The extent to which the task, or social, element of this 'bond' between the group and its members remains a topic of interest for researchers, and similar to the sport, and organisational, psychology literature, the cyberpsychology literature seems to suggest that task needs are somewhat more important in maintaining the online group environment, than are social requirements. For example, Ren et al. (2012) specifically examined the impact of enhancing members' attachment to their online communities, by manipulating levels of group identity or interpersonal bonds. The results of their study revealed that increasing group identity was a more effective way to enhance members' attachment to their online communities, compared to increasing the interpersonal bonds between the members. This implies that members of groups seem to feel a stronger attachment to groups they can relate to more in terms of group objectives and characteristics, rather than those in which they have specifically close-knit social, or attraction-based bonds with other members of the group. Therefore, group identity in online groups appears to fulfil an important function in online group growth and development.

Group and collective identity, roles and norms

The term 'group identity' is a term used to describe the common characteristics and common goals, similar beliefs and standards that often exist between group members (Chen & Li, 2009). 'Collective identity' is a related term which refers to how people are similar to each other within a group, when the psychological connection between the individual self and the social group is considered (Abrams & Hogg, 2001). As with many groups, roles and norms emerge within online groups to allow them to function effectively. A role within any group refers to the 'position' a person may fill within that group, such as a 'leadership' role, similar to a 'captain's role' within a team perhaps. Roles within groups can, therefore, be described as formal or informal. An example of a formal role would be a managerial role or a captaincy role. Such roles are explicitly stated and clearly identified. An informal role could include the 'joker' role, or indeed, the 'peacemaker' role within the group. Norms differ from roles in groups as they typically refer to the rules a group puts in place in order to regulate the behaviour of the group members. Groups often develop their norms by observing the 'normal' or 'accepted' behaviours of other groups (Borsari & Carey, 2003). For example, a norm within a work setting might be that all employees are expected to arrive to work on time, with only special exceptions to this rule being tolerated. Penalties are often put in place to punish members of groups when they 'break' the rules, in order to motivate the members to conform to the group norms, and so that the group can exist in a harmonious way (Kirwan & Power, 2014).

'Depersonalisation' is a specific term within group dynamics used to describe the phenomenon where people conform to a group prototype and behave according to group norms (Code & Zaparyniuk, 2009). At times, in such groups, individuals relinquish their individual views, beliefs or needs, in order to accept the group's views. When individuals find themselves being influenced in such a way by the opinions of other group members, the term 'groupthink' may be used to describe the phenomenon.

Groupthink

As cited above, sometimes a kind of 'groupthink' can emerge in groups. Groupthink refers to changes in the cognitions of individuals in groups, especially when they are in contact with, or interacting with, other group members. The reasons why groupthink occurs has been examined extensively by many social psychologists (Bandura, 1986). Among young people who are likely to join online groups, peer pressure may be one reason why groupthink occurs. In 2008, boyd completed a qualitative study on American teenagers who joined online social networks. boyd reported that strong and direct peer pressure was placed on American teenagers to join online social networks, such as Facebook and Bebo. The teenagers interviewed in boyd's study reported that, in addition to pressure from peers to join these groups, they also experienced feelings of isolation and being 'left out' if they did not join such online communities.

Perhaps different types of online groups are also more, or less, susceptible to features such as groupthink? Researchers have attempted to characterise and generalise online group topographies (Bargh & McKenna, 2004). A limitation of this research has emerged, namely, whether different online groups communicate and interact in similar ways that makes them comparable, or is it possible that they differ significantly in the way they function? Howard (2014) attempted to address this limitation of some of the previous research examining online group formation and function (Bargh & McKenna, 2004), which had, overall, failed to examine the generalisability of online group features identified, such as group identity and social support issues. Howard (2014) specifically examined some of the overlapping qualities of online groups previously identified by researchers such as McKenna and colleagues (see Bargh & McKenna, 2004), qualities such as group identity, social support, self-presentation and well-being. Howard compared three types of online groups, namely a cancer support group (representing an online 'support group'), a Harry Potter fan group (representing an online 'avocation group') and a Lesbian Gay Bisexual Transgender (LGBT) group (representing a 'stigmatised group'). All three groups selected represented forum online groups only. The decision to include such groups alone was made in an attempt to maintain consistency in the comparisons made between the three types of online groups examined. Howard's results indicated that online groups do indeed appear to differ in their properties, especially in relation to their group members' group identity, social support and well-being features. Howard suggested that future research might attempt to uncover *why* group members vary in their characteristics across different types of online groups. Perhaps such research could also shed some light on the reasons why features, such as groupthink, emerge among some online groups more than others.

Of course, group formation and function is influenced by many other factors. One such factor could be the leadership structure within groups, which will now be discussed in relation to online groups.

Leadership roles in online groups

Formal leadership roles have often been examined in the offline world (Moran, 2012). Based on the social identity theory of leadership (Hogg & Reid, 2001), individuals who exhibit more prototypical characteristics of a group typically emerge as the group's leaders. Such individuals often exhibit a high degree of overlap between their own characteristics and the characteristics of the other group members (especially in relation to their goals, values and attitudes). While such incidences apply in the offline world, they could apply more strongly on the Internet where other influential factors for leadership are not as apparent, such as physical appearance and the degree of interpersonal dominance potential leaders might have over other group members (Hogg & Reid, 2001). Regarding specific leadership research in online groups, the question of who governs online chat-rooms, for example, has been examined (Bowker & Liu, 2001). However, overall, this area does not appear to have been researched in great depth in the past ten years and could now be considered in need of examination by current researchers.

Social loafing

Of course, some negative group interactions also exist in online groups, in the same way as they are present in offline groups, such as social loafing. This term refers to individuals' decreased efforts when they are working together as part of a group, compared to working alone on the task. In the offline world, such behaviour can have a significant negative effect on performance, especially within sporting, and work-based, groups (Moran, 2012). Online, social loafing in groups has been linked to variables such as increased group size (Blair *et al.*, 2005), a finding also reported as groups increased in size in the offline environment (Moran, 2012). Ways to minimise the occurrence of such behaviour while maximising the contributions of group members remains a challenge for online groups, as it does for their offline counterparts.

Having discussed matters related to online group cohesion, group identity and negative aspects of group behaviour, such as groupthink and social loafing, the debate surrounding the ability of the Internet either to strengthen the bonds of groups or diminish face-to-face interactions will now be considered.

There was some concern that online communication platforms would dilute traditional human relations (Arora, 2011). However, research findings from the early 2000s suggested that, rather than weakening social bonds between groups and communities, online communities have the ability to add to the offline relationships enjoyed by members of groups (see Wellman *et al.*, 2002). Such online networks may add new layers of activities to offline groups and can, therefore, enhance their positive group interactions. Later research has also shown that some individuals do prefer and form stronger social bonds with online support group members than they do with offline social group members, especially if they are left unsatisfied with the support they have or are receiving within their offline groups – for example, individuals not happy with health, or medically related, concerns or conditions (Eun Chung, 2013).

FUTURE DIRECTIONS FOR RESEARCH IN ONLINE GROUPS

Having reviewed some key issues related to online groups, their behaviours and advantages for group members, a number of exciting areas for future research have emerged. For example, more research on the characteristics of members attracted to different types of online groups is a potential area for future research, as advocated by Howard (2014). More specific research examining the characteristics of online leaders is also warranted, to follow up on research by the likes of Bowker and Liu (2001). Such research could help to increase the number of female leaders in the offline world also – for example, where female representation in power positions remains low, compared to their male counterparts (United Nations (UN) Women, 2014).

CONCLUSION

To conclude, this chapter has given an overview of groups online, what they are, why and how they exist, what their strengths and weaknesses are for group members, and how their continued study may contribute to the overall understanding of group dynamics, both in the online and offline world.

ACTIVITY

Create an online social support network group (on Facebook or Twitter) for young adolescents, focusing on a topical issue, such as cyberbullying or mental health issues (e.g. suicide prevention). Document in a final report all activity on the site, such as the material posted, the membership numbers, the volume of traffic to the site and an analysis of the comments posted on the site.

DISCUSSION QUESTIONS

1 Compare and contrast the behaviours of groups in online and offline environments.
2 Discuss the increasing use of the Internet as a source of social support for group members.
3 Outline the dangers of an over-reliance on social networks, such as Facebook, Twitter and chat-rooms, for primary social support.
4 Discuss the impact of individuals experimenting with their social identity online, both for the individual and the group as a whole.

RECOMMENDED READING LIST

Lina Eklund's study examined the link between online/offline group interactions, using social online gaming. The findings of the study demonstrate how on-and offline interactions are closely linked.

> Eklund, L. (2014). Bridging the online/offline divide: The example of digital gaming. *Computers in Human Behaviour.* DOI: 10.1016/j.chb.2014.06.018.

Howard's study set out to examine the dynamics of three different online groups: a cancer support group, an LGBT forum and a Harry Potter fan forum. The results indicate that such groups do differ in their properties, such as their group members' group identity.

> Howard, M.C. (2014). An epidemiological assessment of online groups and a test of a typology: What are the (dis)similarities of the online group types? *Computers in Human Behavior, 31,* 123–133.

This textbook is a comprehensive source of information on social aspects of the Internet. It provides detail on both the positive and negative influences of the online world.

> Amichai-Hamburger, Y. (2013). *The Social Net: Understanding Our Online Behaviour.* (2nd edn). Oxford: Oxford University Press.

GLOSSARY

Collective identity   Describes how people are similar to each other, when the psychological connection between the individual self and the social group the individual is a member of is considered.

Groupthink   'The tendency for cohesive groups to become so concerned about group consolidation that they fail to critically and realistically evaluate their decisions and antecedent assumptions' (Park, 1990, p. 229).

Group norms   The rules individuals are expected to obey as members of a particular group.

Group roles   The parts that individuals play within a group, or the positions they fill within a group (formal or informal).

Social loafing   Describes the reduction in effort exerted by some individuals when they are performing as part of groups.

REFERENCES

Abrams, D. & Hogg, M.A. (2001). Collective identity: Group membership and self-conception. In M.A. Hogg & S. Tinsdale (eds), *Blackwell Handbook of Social Psychology: Group Processes* (pp. 425–460). Malden, MA: Blackwell.

Arora, P. (2011). Online social sites as virtual parks: An investigation into leisure online and offline. *The Information Society, 27*, 113–120.

Bandura, A. (1986). *Social Foundations of Thought and Action*. Englewoods Cliffs, NJ: Prentice-Hall.

Bargh, J.A. & McKenna, K.Y.A. (2004). The Internet and social life. *Annual Review of Psychology, 55*, 573–590.

Baumeister, R.F. & Leary, M.R. (1995). The need to belong: Desire for interpersonal attachments as a fundamental human motivation. *Psychological Bulletin, 117*(3), 497–529.

Blair, C.A., Thompson, L.F. & Wuensch, K.L. (2005). Electronic helping behaviour: The virtual presence of others makes a difference. *Basic and Applied Social Psychology, 27*, 171–178.

Borsari, B. & Carey, K.B. (2003). Descriptive and injunctive norms in college drinking: A meta-analytic integration. *Journal of Studies on Alcohol and Drugs, 64*(3), 331–341.

Bowker, N.I. & Liu, J.L. (2001). Are women occupying positions of power online? Demographics of chat room operators. *CyberPsychology and Behavior, 4*(5), 631–644.

boyd, d. (2008). Taken out of context: American teen sociality in networked publics. Ph.D. dissertation. University of California-Berkeley, School of Information.

Brunet, P.M. & Schmidt, L.A. (2008). Are shy adults really bolder online? It depends on the context. *CyberPsychology & Behavior, 11*(6), 707–709.

Castelnuovo, G., Gaggioli, A., Mantovani, F. & Riva, G. (2003). From therapy to e-therapy: The integration of traditional techniques and new communication tools in clinical settings. *CyberPsychology & Behavior, 6*(4), 375–382.

Chen, Y. & Li, X. (2009). Group identity and social preferences. *American Economic Review, 99*(1), 431–457.

Chiu, P.Y., Cheung, C.M.K. & Lee, M.K.O. (2008). Online social networks: why do 'we' use Facebook? *Communications in Computer and Information Science, 19*, 67–74.

Chmiel, A., Sienkiewicz, J., Thelwall, M., Paltoglou, G., Buckley, K., Kappas, A. & Holyst, J.A. (2011). Collective emotions online and their influence on community life. *PLoSONE, 6*(7), e22207.DOI: 10.1371/journal.pone.0022207.

Code, J.R. & Zaparyniuk, N. (2009). Social identities, group formation, and the analysis of online communities. In S. Hatzipanagos & S. Warburton (eds), *Handbook of Research on Social Software and Developing Communities Ontologies* (pp. 86–101). Hershey, PA: Ideal Group.

Daneback, K., Månsson, S. & Ross, M.W. (2012). Technological advancements and Internet sexuality: Does private access to the Internet influence online sexual behaviour? *CyberPsychology, Behavior & Social Networking, 15*(8), 386–390.

Ebeling-Witte, S., Frank, M.L. & Lester, D. (2007). Shyness, Internet use, and personality. *CyberPsychology and Behavior, 10*(5), 713–716.

Eklund, L. (2014). Bridging the online/offline divide: The example of digital gaming. *Computers in Human Behaviour.* DOI: 10.1016/j.chb.2014.06.018.

Eun Chung, J. (2013). Social interaction in online support groups: Preference for online social interaction over offline social interaction. *Computers in Human Behaviour, 29*, 1408–1414.

Facebook. (2012). One billion people on Facebook. Retrieved from: http://newsroom.fb.com/News/One-Billion-People-on-Facebook-1c9.aspx.

Gentzler, A.L., Oberhauser, A.M., Westerman, D. & Nadorff, D.K. (2011). College students' use of electronic communication with parents: Links to loneliness, attachment, and relationship quality. *CyberPsychology, Behavior, and Social Networking, 14*(1–2), 71–74.

Hogg, M.A. & Reid, S.A. (2001). Social identity, leadership, and power. In A.Y. Lee-Chai & J.A. Bargh (eds), *The Use and Abuse of Power: Multiple Perspectives on the Causes of Corruption* (pp. 159–180). Philadelphia, PA: Psychology Press.

Howard, M.C. (2014). An epidemiological assessment of online groups and typology: What are the (dis)similarities of the online group types? *Computers in Human Behavior, 31*, 123–133.

Kalpidou, M., Costin, D. & Morris, J. (2011). The relationship between Facebook and the wellbeing of undergraduate college students. *CyberPsychology, Behavior, and Social Networking, 14*(4), 183–189.

Kim, J., LaRose, R. & Peng, W. (2009). Loneliness as the cause and the effect of problematic Internet use: The relationship between Internet use and psychological well-being. *CyberPsychology and Behavior, 12*, 451–455.

Kirwan, G. & Power, A. (2014). What is cyberpsychology? In A. Power & G. Kirwan (eds), *Cyberpsychology and New Media: A Thematic Reader* (pp. 3–14). Hove: Psychology Press.

Kuss, D.J. & Griffiths, M.D. (2011). Online social networking and addiction – a review of the psychological literature. *International Journal of Environmental Research & Public Health, 8*, 3528–3552.

Lewis, S.P. & Arbuthnott, A.E. (2012). Searching for thinspiration: The nature of Internet searches for pro-eating disorder website. *Cyberpsychology, Behavior and Social Networking, 15*(4), 200–204.

Maslow, A.M. (1943). A theory of motivation. *Psychological Review, 50*, 370–396.

McKenna, K.Y.A., Green, A.S. & Gleason, M.E.J. (2002). Relationship formation on the Internet: What's the big attraction? *Journal of Social Issues, 58*, 9–31.

Melville, K. (2010). Facebook use associated with depression. Retrieved from: www.science agogo.com/news/201001022311001data_trunc_sys.shtml.

Moran, A.P. (2012). *Sport and Exercise Psychology: A Critical Introduction*. Hove: Routledge.

Murgado-Armenteros, E.M., Torres-Ruiz, F.J. & Vega-Zamora, M. (2012). Differences between online and face to face focus groups, viewed through two approaches. *Journal of Journal of Theoretical and Applied Electronic Commerce Research*, 7, 73–86. DOI: 10.4067/S0718–18762012000200008

Park, W. (1990). A review of research on groupthink. *Journal of Behavioral Decision Making*, 3(3), 229–245.

Parks, M.R. & Floyd, K. (1995 May). Friends in cyberspace: Exploring personal relationships formed through the Internet. Paper presented at the annual meeting of the International Communication Association, Albuquerque, NM.

Ren, Y., Harper, F.M., Drenner, S., Terveen, L., Kiesler, S., Riedl, J. & Kraut, R.E. (2012). Building member attachment in online communities: Applying theories of group identity and interpersonal bonds. *MIS Quarterly*, 36(3), 841–864.

Riva, G. (2002). The sociocognitive psychology of computer-mediated communication: The present and future of technology-based interactions. *CyberPsychology and Behaviour*, 5(6), 581–598.

Sheldon, K.M., Abad, N. & Hinsch, C. (2011). A two-process view of Facebook use and relatedness need-satisfaction: Disconnection drives use and connection rewards it. *Journal of Personality and Social Psychology*, 100(4), 766–775. DOI:10.1037/a0022407.

Tierney, S. (2006). The dangers and draw of online communication: Pro-anorexia websites and their implications for users, practitioners, and researchers. *Eating Disorders*, 14, 181–190.

United Nations (UN) Women. (2014). Progress for women in politics, but the glass ceiling remains firm. Retrieved from: www.unwomen.org/en/news/stories/2014/3/progress-for-women-in-politics-but-glass-ceiling-remains-firm.

Van Belleghem, S., Thys, D. & De Ruyck, T. (2012). Social media around the world 2012. Retrieved from: www.slideshare.net/InSitesConsulting/social-media-around-the-world-2012-by-insitesconsulting.

Wallace, P.M. (1999). *The Psychology of the Internet*. New York: Cambridge University Press.

Walther, J.B. (2007). Selective self-presentation in Computer Mediated communication: Hyperpersonal dimensions of technology, language and cognition. *Computers in Human Behaviour*, 23, 2538–2557.

Wellman, B., Boase, J. & Chen, W. (2002). The networked nature of community: Online and offline. *IT & Society*, 1(1), 151–165.

5

BELONGING IN AN AGE OF TECHNOLOGY

Kelly-Ann Allen

As a society, while many of us have the ability to connect to more and more people in an increasing variety of ways, the decline in face-to-face communication also means that fewer social opportunities are available for some of those who rely on more traditional forms of interactions (Drago, 2015). Are these changes affecting our social satisfaction and leading to increases in the number of people feeling lonely? Are our social skills suffering as a result? Less-direct exposure to other people and fewer opportunities to experience and observe them at first hand could have a particularly large impact on young people (Goodman-Deane et al., 2016). The connections we have today with family, friends and neighbours are unavoidably shaped by rapid developments in technology. But is technology helping or hampering our sense of belonging? This chapter engages with this question and discusses new research into how rapid changes in technology are influencing our social interactions and sense of belonging.

WHEN TECHNOLOGY DIVIDES

On the 14 March 2019, a 28-year-old shooter opened fire on worshipers at two mosques in Christchurch, New Zealand, leaving 50 people dead and scores of others injured. Technology played a central role in these horrifying events. Not only did the shooter livestream the shootings via Facebook, but he also used other social media sites, including Instagram and Twitter, to post videos, articles and Internet memes that pedalled a toxic far-right agenda of social exclusion and hatred. A manifesto for his actions, criticising racial integration and migration, also circulated online. One of the most disturbing outcomes was the amplification of his message by news and media outlets who broadcast the video stream in the wake of the event, giving his views and actions a global reach that they would have otherwise lacked.

Technology is no longer just an extension of our lives, like a porch built onto a house. It now forms the bricks and mortar of our daily existence. Technology is integrated with all manner of typical behaviours and is used as part of our everyday habits. It intersects our relationships and has an inevitable impact on human development. Children now grow up in environments in which their parents spend far more time in front of screens than did previous generations. Work and domestic labours have always drawn the attention of parents away from their children, but modern technology poses a host of new challenges. Not only does it encourage an "always-on" attitude towards working practices, bringing the workplace home into more households than ever before, but the feed of alerts, texts, message group responses, social media updates, news stories and so on being constantly fed directly into the hands of adults provides additional distractions.

This new environment throws up a range of important questions. What is the impact on children of parents checking their work emails while their child plays alone? How does additional parental screen time affect the social development of children? Are effects compounded if the children are also watching a screen at the same time? Tempting as it is to respond to these questions based on intuitions about negative consequences, it is important to let the research speak for itself. In fact, there do seem to be at least some positive outcomes for parent–child relationships from the increasing prevalence of technology, especially with respect to flexibility with work for some, which may mean more time spent at home. Nevertheless, it seems that parental screen time may indeed have an influence on the amount of time that children spend on their screens, with some studies finding a correlation between parents who spend a lot of time on screen media and children who do likewise (Lauricella et al., 2015).

Screen time also appears to be connected to socioeconomic status. Children from more affluent backgrounds are reportedly using screens less, while children from lower-income families are spending more time on screens (Tandon et al., 2012). This raises the troubling question of whether the excessive use of technology might become responsible for creating yet another disadvantage for those from less affluent backgrounds.

HOW MUCH SCREEN TIME DO PARENTS HAVE OUTSIDE WORK ON AVERAGE?

Parents report as spending as many as nine to 11 hours on screen media each day, with over 80% of that time related to personal use. While this number may seem extremely high, it becomes easier to comprehend when we consider the extent to which we are surrounded by screens in our everyday lives. Not only do most of us carry smartphones, but almost everywhere we go there are also tablets, computers and televisions within easy reach. We do not just use these devices when we are sitting still either – they are constant companions on the go as well, and we have come to rely on them for everything from mapping a journey in our car to summoning up a recipe in the kitchen. We text partners and friends as we walk, and we use email to let people know when we are running late. We may not all be using our devices constantly for nine or more hours each day, but many of us are using them much more than we might first think.

You do not need to look too far afield to find research that raises concerns about the heavy use of electronic devices and the consequent high number of hours of screen time. Studies have identified issues related to a range of negative outcomes for children, such as increases in attention-seeking behaviour, sleep disturbances, language delays, and physical inactivity and impediments to executive functioning, social skill development and school readiness (Richards et al., 2010; Parent et al., 2016; Duch et al., 2013; Christofaro et al., 2016). Technology effects the way we socialise, and this influences how we bond with others and develop a sense of belonging.

WHAT EFFECT CAN SCREEN TIME HAVE ON CHILDREN'S SENSE OF BELONGING WITH THEIR PARENTS?

On the one hand, technology affords us a range of benefits, such as the ability to work remotely or from home, which hold out the possibility of more family-friendly lives. But these potential benefits also come with consequences. While it may please some to work at home surrounded by their family, many others feel additional burdens from increased expectations and demands associated with the assumption that they are available 24/7, and there are in turn inevitable distractions from family and home life. For some, at least, being able to spend more time at home does not equate with having more time for family life. In addition to work burdens, distractions caused by digital media, and particularly smartphones, can often interrupt moments that have the potential for allowing genuine connections between parents and children (Kushlev & Dunn, 2018).

Studies have demonstrated that parents feel less connected to their children the more that parents use their smartphones (Kushlev & Dunn, 2018). Other research has shown that a sense of connection can be interrupted during parent–child learning experiences, with negative consequences for learning outcomes. Indeed, it is easy to see why incidental learning opportunities could easily be hampered by the parent's attention being divided between their child and their smartphone. Unsurprisingly, some children have reported feeling that they actually have to compete against a smartphone for their parents' attention (McDaniel & Radesky, 2018). This issue can be particularly challenging for parents who juggle multiple roles.

ARE THERE ANY POSITIVE EFFECTS OF PARENTAL SCREEN TIME?

At the most basic level, when electronic devices and screen time are used as tools to improve work efficiency and thus free up time to connect and foster relationships with their children, they have a clear, indirect positive effect. But there are also more direct contexts in which benefits can be detected.

CHILD-CENTRED PROGRAMMES

Significant positive effects can also emerge from screen media, and these can make it hard to offer straightforward guidelines about appropriate levels of screen time. For example, there is evidence to suggest that from around two years of age, age-appropriate television programmes that are conscientiously constructed can have educational benefits and provide increased learning opportunities (Mares & Pan, 2013). This has been found to be especially true for programmes that encourage imaginative/pretend play.

VIEWING TOGETHER

Some benefits also derive from parental guidance during a child's interaction with screen media (e.g. when parents view and interact with screen media together with their child). In the case of appropriately guided interactions, research has found some degree of benefit for the promotion of early literacy skills (Strouse et al., 2013). There is also an emerging body of literature that supports the value of certain wellbeing apps on smartphones and tablets, which can help teach children a range of skills related to coping and emotional regulation (Morris et al., 2010; Bakker & Rickard, 2018). However, how these benefits relate specifically to a sense of belonging to family relationships is a question that requires further research.

Other examples of the use of electronic devices can also create moments of meaningful connection, especially when the screen is shared and/or used as a relationship-building tool. A parent's talking and reminiscing with their child over baby photos on a smartphone is just one example of the productive and positive use of screen media. In many cases, context is key to whether an interaction will be an opportunity to build belonging or whether it will distract from belonging.

ADOLESCENTS AND TECHNOLOGY

Once upon a time, not that long ago, adolescents would sit glued to fixed-line telephones, to the great frustration of their parents and anyone trying to call. These days, however, it seems that written communication is preferred over verbal communication. Some analysis of modern communications suggests that written communications are going through a process of rapid change and condensation. In the context of a text, email or instant message, brevity is often key; whole sentences are sometimes reduced to a few consonants and vowels, and words are often done away with entirely in favour of an acronym, symbol or emoji. And while this way of communicating is efficient, we have to wonder whether this style of communicating for young people is allowing them to build the connections they need to fulfil their need to belong and equip them with the necessary skills to build relationships with others in the future.

The effects of technology on adolescent wellbeing may not be as severe as the media frequently leads us to believe (Orben & Przybylski, 2018). However, caution is necessary here: the research is still catching up with contemporary habits, and we do not yet have the kind of data that will allow us to understand the true implications of technology on our sense of belonging to others and to groups. There is already a broad intuitive awareness among the public that the effects of technology can be profound, and this has led more and more people to experiment with the idea of the "digital detox". Increasing numbers of apps are now available to block or limit the use of social media sites, while other tools, such as greyscale filters, can be used to make screen time less appealing. More direct measures can also be taken, with some schools going as far as to enact complete bans on the use of mobile phones on their grounds.

We know that excessive screen time or the compulsion to check our phones for updates can disrupt our ability to connect with others. However, the long-term implications for adolescents on their changing behavioural patterns have not yet been determined. But it is not all doom and gloom. While some of the consequences of modern technology may have concerning implications for the average teenager, even the dangers have the potential to make us more aware of how young people connect with others. For instance, simply reflecting on what we risk losing can lead us to focus more consciously on vital elements of a relationship – especially between parent/caregiver and a young person or the relationships between teenagers.

Another concern that has been raised about the effects of digital technology on young people is the potential of technology to reduce opportunities for the attainment and development of social skills. Turkle (2011) suggests that connecting with people through technological rather than physical means may result in a loss of the types of social skills required for face-to-face interaction. It is reasonable to expect that children who spend large amounts of time on electronic devices could have more social difficulties during later adolescence.

In the absence of research on the topic, many schools have banned the use of mobile phones during class and break times, and some have banned their use on school grounds altogether. These decisions have polarised the academic community, some of whom believe that in the absence of electronic devices, young people will not learn the necessary skills to use them appropriately. School leaders and teachers have anecdotally reported that students are spending less time looking at their devices and more time interacting with peers. What happens beyond the school gates, however, is not under the direct control of schools.

THE BROADER ISSUE

In *Bowling Alone: The Collapse and Revival of American Community*, Robert D. Putnam (2000) writes that the connections we have with family, friends and neighbours are shaped by rapid developments in technology. Putman notes a decline in *social capital* – that is, the value of social networks that arise from social intercourse with other individuals and families. Putman acknowledges that the Internet is a useful tool for connecting *physically distant* people. However, he also asks whether access to technology might challenge the possibility of forming genuine relationships and building communities: "is virtual social capital itself a contradiction of terms?" (p. 170). And he asks whether technology has contributed to a trend in deteriorating social connectedness. These questions were prescient when he wrote his book 20 years ago and have become ever more urgent in the years since. While there is a consensus that feeling a sense of belonging has a positive impact on physical health and wellbeing, further investigation is needed to help us understand the factors which influence belonging itself, particularly with respect to technology.

A MODERN SENSE OF COMMUNITY

A sense of community in the modern world need not be limited by physical contact or geography. Some relational communities are not linked to a locality but are based instead on a shared interest or purpose. McMillan and Chavis (1986) describe a psychological sense of community as a "feeling that members have of belonging, a feeling that members matter to one another and to the group, and a shared faith that members' needs will be met through their commitment to be together" (p. 9).

Research into the structures and the processes underlying online communities and groups is growing. Social media enables individuals to find a smaller subset of the broader community which they identify with and to which they feel they belong. Examples can be found in the formation of online groups around a particular hobby or support groups that enable people to come together around a common issue, adversity or diagnosis. However, few researchers have studied whether online communities create the *same type* of belonging that we feel when we connect to groups in the physical world. The qualities and actions of online groups appear to be like those of offline communities, but although social networks share some features of offline communities (e.g. exchanging resources and social support), more research is needed to investigate the full benefits of belonging towards an *online* community group. It may be that online social networks can serve different functions. For example, casual membership in a social networking site to "keep in contact with friends" might provoke different forms of cognition and different effects than would membership in an online support group or forum designed for individuals with cancer.

In late 2017, Katie Gilchrist (@mysenseoftumour), a senior consultant, was diagnosed with an acoustic neuroma brain tumour. In 2019, she underwent surgery and struggled to find the right social support networks online, so she built her own on Instagram. The following is Katie's story:

> When I was first diagnosed, I went looking online for support networks and information others with the same condition had shared. To my surprise, what I found was a web of negativity. As a way of coping (and also to share my story with others) I created an Instagram account and a blog where I have documented my story from day one. Now with a bit of a following, I have created a community of support for not only myself but others with the same condition.

You can read Katie's blog at https://mysenseoftumour.com.

One explanation for Katie's experience may be that different platforms provide different benefits. Pittman and Reich (2016) found that image-based visual platforms such as Instagram and Snapchat have users with less self-reported loneliness and increased happiness than users of more *text-based* platforms. It may be possible that when we view other photos of people, we are more likely to have the feeling that another person, a friend, is really there.

PERCEPTION OF FRIENDSHIP

Turkle (2011) has suggested that the difference between online communities and offline communities may be rooted in the fact that connecting with people over the Internet gives us only the perception of friendship; we are in contact but we remain physically alone. Jones (1997) suggests that some online groups are *virtual communities*, whereas others are *virtual settlements*, with frequent changes in members and consequently less emotional connection. Researchers have also noted that "heavy Internet use" can alienate people and reduce social contact (e.g. Beard, 2002; Erdoğan, 2008; Weiser, 2001), thereby hindering face-to-face relationships, regardless of the possible value of online communities.

Other scholars have used cross-cultural perspectives to examine perceptions of friendships. Sheldon and colleagues (2017) compared Croatian users and American users of Instagram, finding that Croatian participants reported greater gratification from social media use than did the American participants in the study. The researchers speculated that Croatians were more "we"-focused and Americans more "me"-focused, drawing from individualism vs collectivism thoughts; however, it was also suggested that the Croatian participants perceived their "followers" as friends, whereas American participants were more likely to consider them as "fans".

LONELINESS AND TECHNOLOGY

A major concern that has been raised with the increasing prevalence of technology is its negative association with loneliness. Stepanikova and colleagues (2010) examined digital tools and found that people who spent increased time on the Internet – using chat rooms, messaging groups and newsgroups, for example – felt lonelier than those who spent less time or no time at all. Email neither increased nor decreased wellbeing. While certain studies have shown that the Internet increases loneliness (e.g. Erdoğan, 2008), not all studies have drawn the same conclusion, particularly when investigating certain groups of people. For example, the Internet has actually been shown to decrease feelings of loneliness in people who identify themselves as lonely or shy. Bonetti and colleagues (2010) found that Internet use allowed people who were shy to interact in ways they would not have done in "real life" due to feeling too intimidated. Online groups may, then, provide communities in which shy people can feel emotionally safe.

Studies have also found that people who report feeling lonely may benefit from Internet use, with the research suggesting that increased Internet use can decrease feelings of loneliness and increase social support in real life. Studies have arrived at similar findings when examining Internet use in older and isolated populations (e.g. Khosravi et al., 2016), and people who are considered introverts (Kircaburun & Griffiths, 2018). Kuss and Griffiths (2011) found that extraverts use online platforms to consolidate friendships that already exist, whereas introverts use online networks to create meaningful relationships. There have been further speculations about why social media use may decrease loneliness. Yang (2016) suggests that not all social media use is as passive as it may first appear. In fact, people may use social media as a prelude to social contact. Moreover, social media networks might also remind people about how big their social networks are, even if they are not interacting with them daily.

FINAL THOUGHTS

Given the prevalence of technology in our daily lives, it has never been more important to study its capacity to foster belonging. Research so far has suggested that whether technology detracts from or strengthens our ability to belong is dependent on the context, use and the individual. New technologies change the way we share and consume knowledge but also influence how we socially interact. To really grasp the ongoing effects this kind of technological change has on individuals and society, new research is needed to study not only how the technology itself influences our social interactions and how, in turn, we define belonging, community and advancement but also how we manage and process the speed of the change, the rapid turnover of technologies and the social and cultural change it brings.

REFERENCES

Bakker, D., & Rickard, N. (2018). Engagement in mobile phone app for self-monitoring of emotional wellbeing predicts changes in mental health: Mood-Prism. *Journal of Affective Disorders, 227*, 432–442.

Beard, K. W. (2002). Internet addiction: Current status and implications for employees. *Journal of Employment Counseling, 39*(1), 2–11.

Bonetti, L., Campbell, M. A., & Gilmore, L. (2010). The relationship of loneliness and social anxiety with children's and adolescents' online communication. *Cyberpsychology, Behavior, and Social Networking, 13*(3), 279–285.

Christofaro, D. G. D., De Andrade, S. M., Mesas, A. E., Fernandes, R. A., & Farias Junior, J. C. (2016). Higher screen time is associated with overweight, poor dietary habits and physical inactivity in Brazilian adolescents, mainly among girls. *European Journal of Sport Science, 16*(4), 498–506.

Drago, E. (2015). The effect of technology on face-to-face communication. *Elon Journal of Undergraduate Research in Communications, 6*(1), 13–19.

Duch, H., Fisher, E. M., Ensari, I., Font, M., Harrington, A., Taromino, C., Yip, J., & Rodriguez, C. (2013). Association of screen time use and language development in Hispanic toddlers: A cross-sectional and longitudinal study. *Clinical Pediatrics, 52*(9), 857–865.

Erdoğan, Y. (2008). Exploring the relationships among internet usage, internet attitudes and loneliness of Turkish adolescents. *Cyberpsychology: Journal of Psychosocial Research on Cyberspace, 2*(2), article 4.

Goodman-Deane, J., Mieczakowski, A., Johnson, D., Goldhaber, T., & Clarkson, P. J. (2016). The impact of communication technologies on life and relationship satisfaction. *Computers in Human Behavior, 57*, 219–229.

Jones, Q. (1997). Virtual-communities, virtual settlements & cyber-archaeology: A theoretical outline. *Journal of Computer-Mediated Communication, 3*(3), JCMC331.

Khosravi, P., Rezvani, A., & Wiewiora, A. (2016). The impact of technology on older adults' social isolation. *Computers in Human Behavior, 63*, 594–603. Retrieved from: https://doi.org/10.1016/j.chb.2016.05.092; https://www.sciencedirect.com/science/article/pii/S0747563216304289

Kircaburun, K., & Griffiths, M. D. (2018). Instagram addiction and the Big Five of personality: The mediating role of self-liking. *Journal of Behavioral Addictions, 7*(1), 158–170.

Kushlev, K., & Dunn, E. W. (2019). Smartphones distract parents from cultivating feelings of connection when spending time with their children. *Journal of Social and Personal Relationships*, 36(6), 1619–1639.

Kuss, D. J., & Griffiths, M. D. (2011). Online social networking and addiction – A review of the psychological literature. *International Journal of Environmental Research and Public Health*, 8(9), 3528–3552.

Lauricella, A. R., Wartella, E., & Rideout, V. J. (2015). Young children's screen time: The complex role of parent and child factors. *Journal of Applied Developmental Psychology*, 36, 11–17.

Mares, M. L., & Pan, Z. (2013). Effects of sesame street: A meta-analysis of children's learning in 15 countries. *Journal of Applied Developmental Psychology*, 34(3), 140–151.

McDaniel, B. T., & Radesky, J. S. (2018). Technoference: Longitudinal associations between parent technology use, parenting stress, and child behavior problems. *Pediatric Research*, 84(2), 210–218.

McMillan, D. W., & Chavis, D. M. (1986). Sense of community: A definition and theory. *Journal of Community Psychology*, 14(1), 6–23.

Morris, M. E., Kathawala, Q., Leen, T. K., Gorenstein, E. E., Guilak, F., DeLeeuw, W., & Labhard, M. (2010). Mobile therapy: Case study evaluations of a cell phone application for emotional self-awareness. *Journal of Medical Internet Research*, 12(2), e10.

Orben, A., & Baukney-Przybylski, A. K. (2018). Screens, teens and psychological well-being: Evidence from three time-use diary studies. *Psychological Science*, 30(5), 682–696.

Parent, J., Sanders, W., & Forehand, R. (2016). Youth screen time and behavioral health problems: The role of sleep duration and disturbances. *Journal of Developmental and Behavioral Pediatrics: JDBP*, 37(4), 277–284.

Pittman, M., & Reich, B. (2016). Social media and loneliness: Why an Instagram picture may be worth more than a thousand Twitter words. *Computers in Human Behavior*, 62, 155–167.

Putnam, R. D. (2000). *Bowling alone: The collapse and revival of American community*. New York, NY: Simon and Schuster.

Richards, R., McGee, R., Williams, S. M., Welch, D., & Hancox, R. J. (2010). Adolescent screen time and attachment to parents and peers. *Archives of Pediatrics & Adolescent Medicine*, 164(3), 258–262.

Sheldon, P., Rauschnabel, P. A., Antony, M. G., & Car, S. (2017). A cross-cultural comparison of Croatian and American social network sites: Exploring cultural differences in motives for Instagram use. *Computers in Human Behavior*, 75, 643–651.

Stepanikova, I., Nie, N. H., & He, X. (2010). Time on the Internet at home, loneliness, and life satisfaction: Evidence from panel time-diary data. *Computers in Human Behavior*, 26(3), 329–338.

Strouse, G. A., O'Doherty, K., & Troseth, G. L. (2013). Effective coviewing: Preschoolers' learning from video after a dialogic questioning intervention. *Developmental Psychology*, 49(12), 2368–2382.

Tandon, P. S., Zhou, C., Sallis, J. F., Cain, K. L., Frank, L. D., & Saelens, B. E. (2012). Home environment relationships with children's physical activity, sedentary time, and screen time by socioeconomic status. *International Journal of Behavioral Nutrition and Physical Activity*, 9(1), 88.

Turkle, S. (2011). *Alone together: Why we expect more from technology and less from each other.* New York, NY: Basic Books.

Weiser, E. B. (2001). The functions of internet use and their social and psychological consequences. *Cyberpsychology & Behavior*, 4(6), 723–743.

Yang, C. C. (2016). Instagram use, loneliness, and social comparison orientation: Interact and browse on social media, but don't compare. *Cyberpsychology, Behavior, and Social Networking*, 19(12), 703–708.

6

HOW DO ONLINE SOCIAL NETWORKS INFLUENCE PEOPLE'S EMOTIONAL LIVES?

Ethan Kross and Susannah Chandhok

The advent of online social networking sites like Facebook have rapidly altered the way human beings interact. With a gentle tap of one's finger, people can share their inner thoughts and feelings with untold numbers of people. A gentle swipe down on one's smartphone reveals a compilation of updates on other people's lives from an endlessly populated newsfeed.

These features of social media aren't restricted to an exclusive set of technophiles; they have been widely embraced by humanity. Indeed, at the time of our writing this chapter, close to 2.8 billion people use social media, a number that is predicted to keep rising (Statista, 2019). Moreover, the average user spends approximately 50 minutes per day on Facebook, Instagram, and Facebook Messenger (Stewart, 2016).

But what consequence—if any—does engaging with these online social networks have on how people feel? When we and our colleagues became curious about this issue in the late 2000s, we did what most researchers do when we become interested in a new topic: we performed a literature review. That's when we came across what we now call *The Puzzle*.

On the one hand, several studies revealed negative cross-sectional associations between self-reported Facebook usage and emotional well-being (Farahani, Kazemi, Aghamohamadi, Bakhtiarvand, & Ansari, 2011; Labrague, 2014; Pantic et al., 2012). But other studies revealed the opposite (Datu, Valdez, & Datu, 2012; Ellison, Steinfield, & Lampe, 2007; Nabi, Prestin, & So, 2013; Valenzuela, Park, & Kee, 2009). Still other work suggested that the relationships between Facebook usage and well-being was more nuanced; it depended on additional factors like individual differences in loneliness (Kim, LaRose, & Peng, 2009) or the number of Facebook friends people had (Manago, Taylor, & Greenfield, 2012). At the end of the literature review, we were left with more questions than answers.

In this chapter, we will review the work that we and others have performed to systematically address this puzzle over the past decade. We begin by providing a brief overview of research on online social network usage and well-being, highlighting the conceptual and methodological challenges that prevented early work from drawing strong inferences about the links between these variables. We will then describe a program of research designed to address these concerns by focusing on the mechanisms underlying how two different types of online social network usage—active versus passive usage—shape the emotional outcomes people experience inside and outside of the laboratory. In addressing these issues, we will focus our discussion predominantly on Facebook, the world's largest online social network, because it has been the focus of the majority of empirical attention. We conclude by discussing (a) how researchers can draw inferences about emotion from "big data" and (b) whether online social networks can be strategically harnessed to promote well-being.

Facebook Use & Well-being: Early Research

Does using Facebook influence people's well-being? Our review of early research that focused on this question revealed two issues that made it difficult to answer. First, nearly all of the studies that had been performed on this issue involved asking participants to self-report how much they used Facebook and how they felt in general. While there is clear value to using trait self-report measures to address certain kinds of questions, concerns about using them to measure people's moment-to-moment behaviors and emotions are well-established (for discussion see Kahneman & Deaton, 2010; Kahneman, Krueger, Schkade, Schwarz, & Stone, 2004). Second, the majority of the studies on this topic had utilized cross-sectional, correlational designs that made it impossible to draw inferences about the causal or likely causal relationship between Facebook use and well-being.

As a first step toward overcoming these limitations, we used experience sampling, a methodology that is widely considered the "gold standard" for assessing in vivo behavior and psychological experiences over time and drawing inferences about the *likely* causal sequence of events between variables (Bolger, Davis, & Rafaeli, 2003; Larson & Csikszentmihalyi, 2014). Specifically, over the course of several months, we text messaged 82 participants five times per day between 10 a.m. and midnight for 14 consecutive days, resulting in a data set consisting of 4,589 observations. Each time we texted participants, we asked them to rate how positive and negative they felt. We also asked them to rate how much they had used Facebook since the last time we texted them. We then examined whether the amount of time participants spent using Facebook systematically predicted changes in how they felt from the start of that period to its end.

Our results indicated that the more participants reported using Facebook during one chunk of time, for example, between 9 a.m. and 11 a.m., the more their positive mood declined over the course of that time period. We also found that the reverse pattern of results was not true—i.e., feeling bad at one moment in time did not predict increases in subsequent usage. It was likewise not moderated by any of the individual differences we assessed—e.g., number of Facebook friends, motivation for using Facebook, perceptions of their Facebook network, gender, self-esteem, loneliness, or depressive symptoms.

Importantly, each time we text messaged participants, we also asked them to rate how much they had interacted with other people directly—i.e., face-to-face or via phone—since the last time we text messaged them, to rule out the possibility that any results we observed might be attributed to general social interaction. In fact, our analyses indicated that interacting with other people directly predicted the exact opposite set of results—the more people reported interacting with other people directly during one time period, the more their positive mood rose from the beginning of that time period to its end (Kross et al., 2013).

The paper reporting these results triggered a number of commentaries (e.g., Bohannon, 2013; Konnikova, 2013). In the exchanges that followed, a key question arose: How does Facebook use undermine subjective well-being? To address this question, we turned our attention to the different ways that people interact with Facebook and how it might differentially influence the way they feel.

Prior research had distinguished between two broad categories of Facebook usage: passive and active usage (Burke, Marlow, & Lento, 2010; Deters & Mehl, 2013; Krasnova, Wenninger, Widjaja, & Buxmann, 2013). Passive usage refers to voyeuristically consuming information on a social media site—e.g., scrolling through one's news feed to peer in on the lives of others without generating information. Active usage, on the other hand, involves producing information on the site and engaging in direct exchanges with others—e.g., chatting, uploading posts and pictures. Going into the next phase of the work, we predicted that passively using Facebook in particular might account for its harmful emotional outcomes.

We based this prediction on the idea that social media allows people to curate the way they present themselves to others to a degree that is not possible in daily life. We human beings, of course, always curate how we present ourselves to others to varying degrees (Goffman, 1956, 1963, 1967. Indeed, across multiple seminal works in sociology, Goffman (1956, 1963, 1967) argued that human beings are driven to present themselves in flattering terms. For example, most people think strategically about what clothing they should wear based on who they are going to interact with later on that day. An important meeting may warrant dress attire, whereas a casual get-together with one's friends calls for more relaxed garb. But on social media, the ability to manage the way we present ourselves to others takes on a new form. It allows us to curate the way we appear to others to a degree that is not possible in daily life. We can add filters to our photos, carefully edit our posts, or even send them to friends for review before sharing. Indeed, one study found that a key reason people use Facebook is to serve self-presentational needs (Nadkarni & Hofmann, 2012).

But what might the emotional consequences of scrolling through a world populated by the most glamorized portraits of other people's lives be? Classic research on social comparisons (Festinger, 1954; Goethals, 1986; Wood, 1996) provides a clear answer to this question: When we are exposed to the unobtainable glorified lives of other people, we engage in upward social comparisons that promote envy and lead us to feel worse (Salovey & Rodin, 1984). As argued by Blanton, Burrows and Regan (this volume) in their chapter on health messages in video games, even exaggerated or "unreal" experience with technology can influence real-world behavior. Thus, even if people are aware that a social media profile is augmented beyond something obtainable in reality, such experiences can still have significant consequences on well-being.

We tested these assumptions over the course of two studies (Verduyn et al., 2015). In the first study, we brought participants into the laboratory and randomly assigned them to use Facebook actively or passively for ten minutes. We then assessed how people felt both immediately after the manipulation and at the end of the day (via an email survey).

Immediately after the active versus passive Facebook use manipulations, participants in the two groups did not differ on how they felt. But by the end of the day, participants in the passive Facebook usage group displayed a significant positive emotion decline compared to both their baseline levels of emotion and the levels of end of the day affect that characterized the active Facebook users. The active Facebook usage condition, in contrast, did not display any changes in how they felt over the course of the three assessments.

But were the emotional well-being declines experienced by the passive Facebook users driven by envy? And would these findings be replicated in a more ecologically valid context? We shifted back to experience sampling to address these questions. Specifically, we repeated the experience sampling protocol that we had used in our initial study (Kross et al., 2013), but this time asked people to rate how much they had used Facebook actively and passively since the last time we text messaged them. We also asked them to rate how envious they felt of others each time we texted them.

Our findings indicated that most of the time that people were using Facebook, they were using it passively. In fact, participants used Facebook passively 50 percent more than they did actively. In retrospect, this finding explained why we observed emotional well-being declines linked with overall Facebook usage in our first study (Kross et al. 2013)—i.e., most of the time people were on Facebook, they were likely using it the harmful way. Critically, longitudinal mediation analyses indicated that passive Facebook usage predicted emotional well-being declines, and it did so by promoting feelings of envy. Conceptually replicating the laboratory results, active Facebook usage once again had no impact on people's emotions.

Together, the results from these initial studies began to paint a portrait that described how using Facebook influenced people's emotional lives; an image suggesting that the majority of the times people use Facebook, they do so passively, which in turn leads people to feel envious and predicts declines in their positive mood over time.

Does Counting Emotion Words Provide a Window into Emotion?

An early challenge to these findings came in 2014 when a group of researchers published a controversial experiment in which they manipulated the percentage of positive and negative emotional words contained in 689,003 Facebook users' news feeds for one week (Kramer, Guillory, & Hancock, 2014).[1] The researchers leading the study were interested in examining emotional contagion on social media—i.e., the idea that emotions could spread across social networks just like diseases are transmitted between people who come into physical contact with each other. They predicted that consuming different amounts of positive (or negative) information on social media should lead people to experience more positive or negative emotions in their own lives. They furthermore suggested that they could index people's emotional states by counting the number of emotion words contained in their Facebook posts.

Kramer and colleagues (2014) tested their prediction by manipulating the amount of positive and negative words contained in participants' Facebook news feeds for one week. As predicted, they observed a statistically significant effect of their manipulation. Participants who were exposed to news feeds that contained more (or less) positive (or negative) words ended up using more (or less) positive (or negative) words in their own news feed. They interpreted these findings in support of their predictions noting, "these results indicate that emotions expressed by others on Facebook influence our own emotions, constituting experimental evidence for massive-scale contagion via social networks" (Kramer et al., 2014).

At first blush, these findings directly contradicted the findings that had accumulated up to that point (Kross et al., 2013; Turkle, 2011; Verduyn et al., 2015; Vogel, Rose, Okdie, Eckles, & Franz, 2015). The results of our studies suggested that consuming positive information in other people's news feeds instigates a social comparison process that leaves people feeling worse, not an emotional contagion process that enhances how good people feel.

However, there was an important difference when characterizing these two lines of work. In prior studies on Facebook and well-being, emotional well-being was indexed by asking participants directly how they felt. Concerns about self-report measures notwithstanding, asking people how they feel remains the standard tool for indexing subjective experiences (Kahneman et al., 2004;

Kahneman & Riis, 2005). In the aforementioned study, however, the authors assumed that counting the number of emotion words contained in participants' online social network posts would provide an equally valid tool for drawing inferences about people's emotional experience. But was this a reasonable assumption? Shortly following the publication of the Kramer study, we noted that there were three reasons to question it.

First, word counting methods fail to take context into account. Consider, for example, the following two statements: "I am feeling so great" and "I am not feeling great." A word-counting algorithm that counts the percentage of positive words contained in each of these statements would produce the same result—20 percent (one out of five words in each statement contains a positive emotion word)—even though the two statements convey opposite meaning.

Second, it is well documented that people tend to self-present on social media in ways that may not be accurate or authentic (Nadkarni & Hofmann, 2012; Walther, Van Der Heide, Ramirez, Burgoon, & Peña, 2015). For example, in response to learning that a colleague received a job promotion, a person might write, "That's great news," but not really feel happy for their colleague. They might also simply try to mimic the person they are interacting with to enhance rapport, a common technique in face-to-face interactions (Chartrand & Bargh, 1999; Chartrand & Jefferis, 2003). Thus, we suggested that it was also possible that a person might say something online that on the surface conveyed positive (or negative) emotion, but didn't correlate with how they actually felt.

Finally, compounding these conceptual concerns was the fact that no validation evidence existed to support the idea that counting emotion words on online social networks does in fact track how people feel. Some studies had looked at the correlation between online social network emotional word usage and judges' ratings of the emotionality of participants' posts. But if participants' posts don't honestly convey how they feel, then there's no reason to expect judges to be able to accurately categorize participants' posts (for additional validation concerns see Kross et al., 2018).

So, do people's usage of emotion words in their posts actually reflect how they feel? To address this question, we collapsed four experience sampling data sets that contained two types of information: (a) participants' self-reports of how they felt throughout the day and (b) their Facebook wall posts corresponding to the same time period that they rated their emotions (Kross et al., 2018). For each participant, we computed the percentage of positive and negative words contained in their posts and then examined whether they correlated with how participants reported feeling around the same time that they made each post. Regardless of how we analyzed the data, our results did not reveal any significant associations between participants' usage of emotion words in their Facebook posts and their self-reports of how they felt—a set of findings that cast doubt on researchers' ability to draw inferences about people's emotional states by counting the number of emotion words contained in their online social network posts (for conceptual replication, see Sun, Schwartz, Son, Kern, & Vazire, in press).

The Broader Landscape

Between 2004 and 2012, 412 studies on Facebook were published. Yet, not a single one of those papers examined the relationship between Facebook usage and changes in people's well-being over time. Since that time, the literature on this topic has grown substantially. In 2017, we reviewed this literature, focusing specifically on longitudinal and experimental studies that had examined the relationship between Facebook usage and well-being up to that point (Verduyn, Ybarra, Résibois, Jonides, & Kross, 2017). We concluded that passive Facebook usage robustly predicts emotional well-being declines whereas the relationship between active Facebook usage and well-being was more tenuous. While some relationships revealed positive links between active Facebook usage and well-being improvements, many studies did not.

Since our 2017 review, several additional large-scale studies have been performed which broadly align with these conclusions. For example, Tromholt (2016) randomly assigned over a thousand Danish participants to either use Facebook as usual, or stop using it altogether. Results indicated that Facebook abstention led to an increase in both cognitive and affective well-being (also see Mosquera, Odunowo, McNamara, Guo, & Petrie, 2018; and Allcott, Braghieri, Eichmeyer, & Gentzkow, 2019).

In 2018, researchers at the University of Pennsylvania adopted a slightly different approach to experimentally examine the effects of online social network usage on emotionality (Hunt, Marx, Lipson, & Young, 2018). Rather than use a deprivation paradigm that cut off participants' Facebook usage entirely, they randomly assigned 143 participants to either keep using social media as usual or to limit social media use to ten minutes per day for three weeks. Their results indicated that the limited social media use group showed significant reductions in loneliness and depression over the course of the study period. However, there were no significant effects on social support, self-esteem, or psychological well-being—a pattern of differential results that points to the need for future research to examine how the nature and length of Facebook interventions may systematically impact different variables (Hunt et al., 2018).

Finally, in one particularly persuasive study, Shakya and Christakis (2017) used Facebook log data in conjunction with three waves of nationally representative data to examine the longitudinal relationship between Facebook usage and changes in well-being over time in a sample of 5,208 participants. Their prospective findings indicated that Facebook use predicted decreases in well-being over time (Shakya & Christakis, 2017). Interestingly, the authors found that the more often participants engaged in active usage behaviors like updating one's status or liking another post, the more likely they were to have lower self-reported well-being—a finding that further speaks to the potentially nuanced nature of the relationship between active social media usage and well-being.

Frequently Asked Questions

Given the prevalence of social media, and the somewhat counterintuitive nature of the findings suggesting that a technology built to connect people frequently ends up undermining rather than elevating their positive mood, it is perhaps not surprising that people often have several questions about the aforementioned findings. Here we address two common questions that often arise.

FAQ #1: Why do people continue to use social media if doing so consistently leads them to feel worse? It is well established that people are motivated to approach pleasure and avoid pain (e.g., Freud, 1920; Higgins, 1997). Given this feature of the human condition, why do people continue to engage in a behavior that undermines their positive mood? Although a definitive answer to this question has yet to emerge, here we suggest three possibilities.

First, human behavior is multiply determined; there are several goals activated at any moment. In the context of social media, for example, we may be motivated to engage in a behavior that improves the way we feel. But we may also be motivated by social goals that motivate us to stay abreast of how our social networks are functioning. In this vein, one study found that 88 percent of people report using social media to maintain social relationships (Whiting & Williams, 2013). Thus, it is possible that people use social media despite its negative emotional effects because doing so allows people to stay informed of what is happening in their social networks.

Second, it is well established that people engage in behaviors that they are addicted to even when they reap negative consequences—a phenomenon that neuroscience research has illuminated by highlighting the fact that different brain systems are involved in *wanting* and *liking* (Robinson & Berridge, 2001). These findings are noteworthy in the current context because a growing amount of evidence suggests that social media has addictive properties (Alter, 2017; Andreassen, 2015; Ryan, Chester, Reece, & Xenos, 2014). Further research could examine the role of desire and motivated behavior in social media use (for more details about real-world applications of this cognitive theory, see Papies, this volume).

Finally, some research suggests that people mispredict how using Facebook will make them feel. For example, one study found that participants predicted they would feel better after using Facebook for 20 minutes. In fact, they felt worse after doing so (Sagioglou & Greitemeyer, 2014). This misprediction might be captured by an evolutionary mismatch between how our brains evolved to seek social connections, and the negative consequences they yield on social media (see van Vugt et al., this volume, for a discussion about the concept of evolutionary mismatches).

Taken together, these different findings begin to explain why people may continue to engage in a behavior that leads to emotional well-being declines. However, future research is needed to examine the role that each of these and other factors play in isolation and interactively in predicting types of social media usage.

FAQ #2: Are there ways of harnessing social media to improve well-being? There are many attempts underway to address this important question. One route that we have pursued to examine this issue involves focusing on people suffering from depression. A large literature stretching back to the 1980s indicates that people with depression are characterized by impoverished social support networks (Fiore, Becker, & Coppel, 1983; Rook, 1984). One of the explanations that research has provided for why individuals with depression are characterized by low social support is because they talk frequently about their negative feelings (Blumberg & Hokanson, 1983; Kuiper & McCabe, 1985) in ways that end up pushing away those that care about them (Teichman & Teichman, 1990). In other words, there may be poor interpersonal synchrony between individuals with depression and others (for more details about interpersonal synchrony, please see Koole et al., this volume).

Park and colleagues (2016) were interested in whether these findings would generalize to social media. Given the psychological distance that social media provides people with, they wondered whether the social networks of depressed individuals might be more responsive in the online versus offline world. They addressed this question across two studies (Park et al., 2016).

In Study 1, they focused on an unselected sample of participants with varying levels of depressive symptoms; in Study 2 they recruited psychiatrically diagnosed individuals with Major Depressive Disorder and their age-matched control participants. Across both studies, the experimenters had judges code how supportive the posts of participants' Facebook friends were in response to any negative experiences described by participants on their Facebook accounts over the course of a month. They then compared the amount of support that depressed versus non-depressed participants received, controlling for the number of negative expressions that participants made during the month-long period. As expected, participants with depression self-disclosed negative information more and positive information less to their Facebook networks. However, in direct contrast to prior research examining the links between offline social support and depression, participants with depression received *more* social support from their Facebook friends.

These findings illustrate how social media may provide a platform for providing social support to individuals that may otherwise have difficulty acquiring it, highlighting the need for future research to extend these findings to other vulnerable populations. In particular, one application of social psychology to this line of research would be in testing which aspects of a social media platform could be manipulated to provide better social support for its members.

Concluding Comment

> The Internet does not, contrary to current popular opinion, have by itself the power or ability to control people, to turn them into addicted zombies, or make them dispositionally sad or lonely ... the Internet is one of several social domains in which an individual can live his or her life, and attempt to fulfill his or her needs and goals, whatever they happen to be.
>
> *McKenna & Bargh, 2000*

At the turn of the millennium, McKenna and Bargh concluded that the overall sentiment toward the internet was negative, if not "apocalyptic" (McKenna & Bargh, 2000). Over the course of the next few years, they documented the beneficial aspects of internet use, highlighting how it can foster social relationships and provide people with meaningful routes to express themselves authentically (Bargh, McKenna, & Fitzsimons, 2002; Bargh & McKenna, 2004).

Their work was notably published before the birth of Facebook in 2004. Since that time, the tide of research has drawn away from focusing on internet use to examining the links between social media and well-being instead. Yet, we see a similar pattern emerging. Some have voiced a concern that digital technology is destroying society (Twenge, 2017). Other have suggested that social networking addiction should be a clinically diagnosable disorder and have developed a Facebook Addiction Scale (Andreassen et al., 2012; Karaiskos et al., 2010; Ryan et al., 2014; also see Alter, 2017).

The goal of this chapter is not to paint a picture one way or the other about social media being good or bad. The social media world is multifaceted. Much like the offline terrestrial world, social media allows people to experience an infinite number of healthy and harmful emotional experiences. A critical challenge for future research is to illuminate the mechanisms that systematically predict these different kinds of emotional experiences. Doing so has the potential to enrich our understanding of how a ubiquitous technology can be harnessed to promote rather than undermine well-being.

Note

1 The controversy was a function of the fact that Facebook users were unaware that they were participating in this experiment (Kosinski, Matz, Gosling, Popov, & Stillwell, 2015; Puschmann & Bozdag, 2014; Shaw, 2016).

References

Allcott, H., Braghieri, L., Eichmeyer, S., & Gentzkow, M. (2019). *The welfare effects of social media.* 116.

Alter, A. (2017). *Irresistible: The rise of addictive technology and the business of keeping us hooked.* New York, NY: Penguin Press.

Andreassen, C. S. (2015). Online social network site addiction: A comprehensive review. *Current Addiction Reports, 2*(2), 175–184. doi.org/10.1007/s40429-015-0056-9

Andreassen, C. S., Torsheim, T., Brunborg, G. S., & Pallesen, S. (2012). Development of a Facebook addiction scale. *Psychological Reports, 110*(2), 501–517.

Bargh, J. A., & McKenna, K. Y. (2004). The Internet and social life. *Annual Review of Psychology, 55,* 573–590.

Bargh, J. A., McKenna, K. Y., & Fitzsimons, G. M. (2002). Can you see the real me? Activation and expression of the "true self" on the Internet. *Journal of Social Issues, 58*(1), 33–48.

Blumberg, S. R., & Hokanson, J. E. (1983). The effects of another person's response style on interpersonal behavior in depression. *Journal of Abnormal Psychology, 92*(2), 196–209. doi.org/10.1037/0021-843X.92.2.196

Bohannon, J. (2013, August 14). ScienceShot: Facebook is making you sad. *Science Magazine.* Retrieved from www.sciencemag.org/news/2013/08/scienceshot-facebook-making-you-sad.

Bolger, N., Davis, A., & Rafaeli, E. (2003). Diary methods: Capturing life as it is lived. *Annual Review of Psychology, 54*(1), 579–616. doi.org/10.1146/annurev.psych.54.101 601.145030

Burke, M., Marlow, C., & Lento, T. (2010, April). Social network activity and social well-being. In *Proceedings of the SIGCHI conference on human factors in computing systems* (pp. 1909–1912). ACM.

Chartrand, T. L., & Bargh, J. A. (1999). The chameleon effect: The perception-behavior link and social interaction. *Journal of Personality & Social Psychology, 76*(6), 893–9101.

Chartrand, T. L., & Jefferis, V. E. (2003). Consequences of automatic goal pursuit and the case of nonconscious mimicry. In J. P. Forgas & K. D. Williams (Eds.), *Social judgments: Implicit and explicit processes* (pp. 290–305). New York: Cambridge University Press.

Datu, J. A. D., Valdez, J. P., & Datu, N. (2012). Does Facebooking make us sad? Hunting relationship between Facebook use and depression among Filipino adolescents. *International Journal of Research Studies in Educational Technology, 1*(2). doi.org/10.5861/ijrset.2012.202

Deters, F. große, & Mehl, M. R. (2013). Does posting Facebook status updates increase or decrease loneliness? An online social networking experiment. *Social Psychological and Personality Science, 4*(5), 579–586. doi.org/10.1177/1948550612469233

Ellison, N. B., Steinfield, C., & Lampe, C. (2007). The benefits of Facebook "friends:" Social capital and college students' use of online social network sites. *Journal of Computer-Mediated Communication, 12*(4), 1143–1168. doi.org/10.1111/j.1083-6101.2007.00367.x

Farahani, H. A., Kazemi, Z., Aghamohamadi, S., Bakhtiarvand, F., & Ansari, M. (2011). Examining mental health indices in students using Facebook in Iran. *Procedia – Social and Behavioral Sciences, 28,* 811–814. doi.org/10.1016/j.sbspro.2011.11.148

Festinger, L. (1954). A theory of social comparison processes. *Human Relations, 7*(2), 117–140. doi.org/10.1177/001872675400700202

Fiore, J., Becker, J., & Coppel, D. B. (1983). Social network interactions: A buffer or a stress. *American Journal of Community Psychology; New York, 11*(4), 423–439.

Freud, S. (1920). Beyond the pleasure principle. In J. Strachey, A. Freud, A. Strachey, & A. Tyson (Trans.), *Beyond the pleasure principle, group psychology and other works (1925-1926)* (pp. 1–64).

Goethals, G. R. (1986). Social comparison theory: Psychology from the lost and found. *Personality and Social Psychology Bulletin, 12,* 261–278. doi.org/10.1177/0146167286123001

Goffman, E. (1956). *The presentation of self in everyday life.* New York, NY: Anchor Books.

Goffman, E. (1963). *Behavior in public places.* New York: Free Press.

Goffman, E. (1967). *Interaction ritual.* New York: Pantheon.

Higgins, E. T. (1997). Beyond pleasure and pain. *American Psychologist, 52*(12), 1280–1300. doi.org/10.1037/0003-066X.52.12.1280

Hunt, M. G., Marx, R., Lipson, C., & Young, J. (2018). No more FOMO: Limiting social media decreases loneliness and depression. *Journal of Social and Clinical Psychology, 37*(10), 751–768. doi.org/10.1521/jscp.2018.37.10.751

Karaiskos, D., Tzavellas, E., Balta, G., & Paparrigopoulos, T. (2010). Social network addiction: A new clinical disorder? *European Psychiatry, 25,* 855.

Kahneman, D., & Deaton, A. (2010). High income improves evaluation of life but not emotional well-being. *Proceedings of the National Academy of Sciences, 107*(38), 16489–16493. doi.org/10.1073/pnas.1011492107

Kahneman, D., & Krueger, A. B., Schkade, D. A., Schwarz, N., & Stone, A. A. (2004). A survey method for characterizing daily life experience: The day reconstruction method. *Science, 306*(5702), 1776–1780. doi.org/10.1126/science.1103572

Kahneman, D., & Riis, J. (2005). Living, and thinking about it: Two perspectives on life. In F. A. Huppert, N. Baylis, & B. Keverne (Eds.), *The science of well-being* (pp. 284–305). doi.org/10.1093/acprof:oso/9780198567523.003.0011

Kim J., LaRose R., Peng, W. (2009). Loneliness as the cause and the effect of problematic Internet use: The relationship between Internet use and psychological well-being. *Cyberpsychology & Behavior: The Impact of the Internet, Multimedia and Virtual Reality on Behavior and Society, 12,* 451–455.

Konnikova, M. (2013, September 10). How Facebook makes us unhappy. *The New Yorker.* Retrieved from www.newyorker.com/tech/annals-of-technology/how-facebook-makes-us-unhappy

Kosinski, M., Matz, S. C., Gosling, S. D., Popov, V., & Stillwell, D. (2015). Facebook as a research tool for the social sciences: Opportunities, challenges, ethical considerations, and practical guidelines. *American Psychologist, 70*(6), 543–556. doi.org/10.1037/a0039210

Kramer, A. D. I., Guillory, J. E., & Hancock, J. T. (2014). Experimental evidence of massive-scale emotional contagion through social networks. *Proceedings of the National Academy of Sciences, 111*(24), 8788–8790. doi.org/10.1073/pnas.1320040111

Krasnova, H., Weminger, H., Widjaja, T., & Buxmann, P. (2013). *Envy on Facebook: A hidden threat to users' life satisfaction?* 11th International Conference on Wirtschaftsinformatik (WI).

Kross, E., Verduyn, P., Boyer, M., Drake, B., Gainsburg, I., Vickers, B., … Jonides, J. (2018). Does counting emotion words on online social networks provide a window into people's subjective experience of emotion? A case study on Facebook. *Emotion, 19,* 97–107. doi.org/10.1037/emo0000416

Kross, E., Verduyn, P., Demiralp, E., Park, J., Lee, D. S., Lin, N., … Ybarra, O. (2013). Facebook use predicts declines in subjective well-being in young adults. *PLoS One*, *8*(8), e69841. doi.org/10.1371/journal.pone.0069841

Kuiper, N. A., & McCabe, S. B. (1985). The appropriateness of social topics: Effects of depression and cognitive vulnerability on self and other judgments. *Cognitive Therapy and Research*, *9*(4), 371–379. doi.org/10.1007/BF01173087

Labrague, L. J. (2014). Facebook use and adolescents' emotional states of depression, anxiety, and stress. *Health Science Journal*, *8*(1), 80–89.

Larson, R., & Csikszentmihalyi, M. (2014). The experience sampling method. In M. Csikszentmihalyi, *Flow and the foundations of positive psychology* (pp. 21–34). doi.org/10.1007/978-94-017-9088-8_2

Manago, A. M., Taylor, T., & Greenfield, P. M. (2012). Me and my 400 friends: The anatomy of college students' Facebook networks, their communication patterns, and well-being. *Developmental Psychology*, *48*(2), 369–380.

McKenna, K. Y., & Bargh, J. A. (2000). Plan 9 from cyberspace: The implications of the Internet for personality and social psychology. *Personality and Social Psychology Review*, *4*(1), 57–75.

Mosquera, R., Odunowo, M., McNamara, T., Guo, X., & Petrie, R. (2018). The economic effects of Facebook. *SSRN Electronic Journal*. doi.org/10.2139/ssrn.3312462

Nabi, R. L., Prestin, A., & So, J. (2013). Facebook friends with (health) benefits? Exploring social network site use and perceptions of social support, stress, and well-being. *Cyberpsychology, Behavior, and Social Networking*, *16*(10), 721–727. doi.org/10.1089/cyber.2012.0521

Nadkarni, A., & Hofmann, S. G. (2012). Why do people use Facebook? *Personality and Individual Differences*, *52*(3), 243–249. doi.org/10.1016/j.paid.2011.11.007

Pantic, I., Damjanovic, A., Todorovic, J., Topalovic, D., Bojovic-Jovic, D., Ristic, S., & Pantic, S. (2012). Association between online social networking and depression in high school students: Behavioral physiology viewpoint. *Psychiatria Danubina*, *24*(1), 90–93.

Park, J., Lee, D. S., Shablack, H., Verduyn, P., Deldin, P., Ybarra, O., … Kross, E. (2016). When perceptions defy reality: The relationships between depression and actual and perceived Facebook social support. *Journal of Affective Disorders*, *200*, 37–44. doi.org/10.1016/j.jad.2016.01.048

Puschmann, C., & Bozdag, E. (2014). Staking out the unclear ethical terrain of online social experiments. *Internet Policy Review*. Retrieved from https://policyreview.info/articles/analysis/staking-out-unclear-ethical-terrain-online-social-experiments

Robinson, T. E., & Berridge, K. C. (2001). Incentive-sensitization and addiction. *Addiction*, *96*(1), 103–114. doi.org/10.1046/j.1360-0443.2001.9611038.x

Rook, K. S. (1984). The negative side of social interaction: Impact on psychological well-being. *Journal of Personality and Social Psychology*, *46*(5), 1097–1108. doi.org/10.1037/0022-3514.46.5.1097

Ryan, T., Chester, A., Reece, J., & Xenos, S. (2014). The uses and abuses of Facebook: A review of Facebook addiction. *Journal of Behavioral Addictions*, *3*(3), 133–148. doi.org/10.1556/JBA.3.2014.016

Sagioglou, C., & Greitemeyer, T. (2014). Facebook's emotional consequences: Why Facebook causes a decrease in mood and why people still use it. *Computers in Human Behavior*, *35*, 359–363. doi.org/10.1016/j.chb.2014.03.003

Salovey, P., & Rodin, J. (1984). Some antecedents and consequences of social-comparison jealousy. *Journal of Personality and Social Psychology*, *47*(4), 780–792. doi.org/10.1037/0022-3514.47.4.780

Shakya, H. B., & Christakis, N. A. (2017). Association of Facebook use with compromised well-being: A longitudinal study. *American Journal of Epidemiology*. doi. org/10.1093/aje/kww189

Shaw, D. (2016). Facebook's flawed emotion experiment: Antisocial research on social network users. *Research Ethics, 12*(1), 29–34. doi.org/10.1177/1747016115579535

Statista. (2019). Number of social media users worldwide from 2010 to 2021 (in billions). Retrieved May 6, 2019 from www.statista.com/statistics/278414/number-of-worldwide-social-network-users/

Stewart, J. B. (2016). Facebook has 50 minutes of your time each day. It wants more. *The New York Times*. Retrieved from http://www.nytimes.com/2016/05/06/business/facebook-bends-the-rules-ofaudience-engagement-to-its-advantage.html. Retrieved October 12, 2016.

Sun, J., Schwartz, H. A., Son, Y., Kern, M. L., & Vazire, S. (in press). The language of well-being: Tracking fluctuations in emotion experience through everyday speech. *Journal of Personality and Social Psychology*.

Teichman, Y., & Teichman, M. (1990). Interpersonal view of depression: Review and integration. *Journal of Family Psychology, 3*(4), 349–367. doi.org/10.1037/h0080549

Tromholt, M. (2016). The Facebook experiment: Quitting Facebook leads to higher levels of well-being. *Cyberpsychology, Behavior, and Social Networking, 19*(11), 661-666.

Turkle, S. (2011). *Alone together: Why we expect more from technology and less from each other*. New York, NY: Basic Books.

Twenge, J. M. (2017, September). Have smartphones destroyed a generation? *The Atlantic*. Retrieved from www.theatlantic.com/magazine/archive/2017/09/ has-the-smartphone-destroyed-a-generation/534198/

Valenzuela, S., Park, N., & Kee, K. F. (2009). Is there social capital in a social network site? Facebook use and college students' life satisfaction, trust, and participation. *Journal of Computer-Mediated Communication, 14*(4), 875–901. doi.org/10.1111/j.1083-6101. 2009.01474.x

Verduyn, P., Lee, D. S., Park, J., Shablack, H., Orvell, A., Bayer, J., … Kross, E. (2015). Passive Facebook usage undermines affective well-being: Experimental and longitudinal evidence. *Journal of Experimental Psychology: General, 144*(2), 480–488. doi.org/10. 1037/xge0000057

Verduyn, P., Ybarra, O., Résibois, M., Jonides, J., & Kross, E. (2017). Do social network sites enhance or undermine subjective well-being? A critical review. *Social Issues and Policy Review, 11*(1), 274–302. doi.org/10.1111/sipr.12033

Vogel, E. A., Rose, J. P., Okdie, B. M., Eckles, K., & Franz, B. (2015). Who compares and despairs? The effect of social comparison orientation on social media use and its outcomes. *Personality and Individual Differences, 86*, 249–256. doi.org/10.1016/j.paid. 2015.06.026

Walther, J. B., Van Der Heide, B., Ramirez, A., Burgoon, J. K., & Peña, J. (2015). Interpersonal and hyperpersonal dimensions of computer-mediated communication. In S. S. Sundar (Ed.), *The handbook of the psychology of communication technology* (pp. 1–22). doi.org/10.1002/9781118426456.ch1

Whiting, A., & Williams, D. (2013). Why people use social media: A uses and gratifications approach. *Qualitative Market Research: An International Journal, 16*(4), 362–369. doi.org/10.1108/QMR-06-2013-0041

Wood, J. V. (1996). What is social comparison and how should we study it? *Personality and Social Psychology Bulletin, 22*, 520–537. doi.org/10.1177/0146167296225009

7 Online relationship formation

Ilan Talmud and Gustavo Mesch

Introduction

As stated in Chapter 3, online sociability is an integral part of young people's digital literacy and cultural consumption of technological artefacts. The ability of the Internet to facilitate online contact, especially with geographically remote people, has caught the popular imagination and the empirical attention of researchers studying online relationship formation. The main consequence of adolescents' online engagement is the expansion of their social ties. However, this expansion is random. It is confined by social regularities governing the ways in which humans interact, online or offline, thus making the formation patterns of online social ties predictable by social analysts.

Studies on the use of ICT by youth apprise us of the active role that youth play in online activity, and that the parents' and the adolescents' views regarding ICT do not always converge. Parents indicate that the computer is bought and connected to the Internet, reflecting their willingness to provide a tool to improve their children's academic performance, to provide access to information needed for school work, to adapt to the school requirement of typed assignments, and to link the teens to the information society. By contrast, teens experience the Internet as a tool for social purpose and play (Lenhart et al., 2001; Livingstone and Bober, 2004; Cohen, Lamish, and Schejter, 2008). Boase and Wellman (2006) argue that in contrast to the popular image of the Internet as a trigger and facilitator of new relationships, "only a relatively small proportion of internet users have ever met someone new online."

Adolescents play an active role in their communicative conduct. Consequently, their primary uses of the Internet do not always match their parents' expectations and wishes. Adolescents are most likely to use the Internet to communicate with others for social and gaming purposes, and in some cases to reach out and communicate with others not of their proximate or immediate social circle at school or in their neighborhood. Moreover, adolescents learn to utilize computer-mediated communication as an additional form of social environment, developing digital literacy, and making new contacts over the Internet. Online relationships nowadays appear to be an integral part of youth culture (Helsper, 2008a). The technological features of ICT smooth barriers of communication, yet they cannot completely remove the effects of social constraints on social interaction. The odds of forming new relations are higher among those socially similar, geographically close, and having at least one friend in common ("transitive relations") (Kadushin, 2004). Forming online relationships might be one of the most appealing aspects of Internet use to young people, given that forming relationships is an important developmental task of adolescence, and in this task youth are limited in their choices by geographical constraints.

Understanding the process involves studying motivations impelling youth to form relationships online, their choice of communication channels and content, the effect of online ties on young people's existing ties and social life, and the quality of online associations. In this chapter, we tackle these topics.

The notion of online relationship formation requires conceptual clarification. Most research has not clearly defined what is meant by online ties. It was largely conducted to elucidate the effects of channel characteristics on interpersonal communication, emphasizing the lack of social presence, lack of richness, and lack of clues in Internet communication (Sproul and Kissler, 1986), and it sought the conditions under which this communication is non-personal or becomes hyper-personal (Walther, 1996). Another direction has been research to understand channel choice across distances and to inquire whether one online communication supplements or replaces the use of other channels of communication among kin and friends. These studies show that Internet use is associated with more and not less communication, and that the more individuals contact by phone and face-to-face, the more they contact using email (Chen et al., 2002); it is suggested that connectivity increases local and long-distance communication (Hampton and Wellman, 2002). Most of this research reflects the conduct of online communication but makes no major attempt to define the nature of the online relationship. Lack of conceptual clarity may lead to contradictory findings.

Prior to the information age, adolescents' social choices were severely restricted by time and place. Their lack of geographical mobility and their belonging to an age group expected to go to school structurally reduced their social circle to friends who were in the neighborhood, at school, and at extracurricular activities. Proximity was a central social constraint for relationship formation. Living in the same neighborhood and attending the same school entailed a high level of social similarity.

Internet and mobile access and communication have produced a number of changes in social communication patterns. Relationship formation has been expanded from geographical spaces of interaction (the neighborhood, the school) to digital spaces (social networks applications). Friendships that in the past were based on social groups with clear boundaries and social expectations of mutual interaction changed to personalized peer-diverse and dispersed personalized peer networks that lack clear boundaries and norms of social behavior. Channels of interpersonal communication are multiplex, including in addition to face-to-face and phone, mobile applications and diverse platforms of social media.

As a result, the limits of interpersonal communication have been blurred and include:

- perpetual contact with the social network anywhere and anytime;
- communication is personalized, relying on ego-networks rather than social groups;
- contents are not exclusive and can be forwarded without the owner's knowledge;
- activities are coordinated through social media.

These major changes in the patterns, frequency, content, and quality in interpersonal friendship formation, maintenance, and communication have been noted by a large number of studies that focus on different aspects of this major social change. In this chapter we focus on one important aspect, namely, the similarities, differences, and overlaps between online and offline social relationships.

With the growing popularity and ubiquity of social media, the public and, to some extent, also research were concerned with the increasing growth of online relationships and the concern that these are replacing more high quality offline relationships. Studies conducted in the early 1990s found that adolescents in western countries were reporting that they meet individuals and maintained interpersonal communication with others whom they had met online at the same time as they met with friends face-to-face. Online/offline relationships were at that time defined according to the space of interaction that the respondents indicated was where they meet their friends. Online relationships were the ones that were formed in forums, chat rooms, gaming, and messenger. Offline relationships were usually defined as the ones that were initiated in the neighborhood, school, or any other face-to-face space of social interaction.

It is important to recognize that a comparison between the two kinds of relationships designated as online and offline may imply either that they are mutually exclusive or opposed to each other. Yet over time is clear that interpersonal relationships are created, developed, and sustained through integrated online and offline interaction. The entire range of offline relationships, from family through school and work to social relations in the wider neighborhood, may also be present online in a manner that is rarely separated out from one's offline life. The popular perception of online relationships as relationships that can be contrasted with a "real world"—inhabited by one's real or more authentic offline relationships—seems therefore simplistic and misleading. This corresponds to an earlier critique of the concept of the "virtual," a term prominent during the early years of Internet use. In short, our study treats social media in much the same way that everyone treats the landline telephone, never described today as a separate "online/on-phone" facet of life. It is, however, essential for us as researchers to recognize that whatever misgivings we may feel as academics about this dualistic terminology, it remains a primary mode by which people around the world understand and experience digital media.

Because of this perception that online life can be contrasted to offline life, we start this chapter with a summary of the perspectives that explain online relationships formation.

"The rich get richer hypothesis" proposes that individuals with higher extroversion, who are more more comfortable in social situations or have already social resources would be more likely to use social media for online relationship formation, extending their social networks and enhancing the quality of their friendships (Kraut et al., 2002). According to this hypothesis, individuals who are extroverted and already have strong social skills would do better in sharing their views and asking for help online, thereby attaining additional social support and higher life satisfaction through cyberspace (Khan et al., 2016).

Conversely, "the poor get poorer hypothesis" argues that individuals who are introverted have higher levels of social anxiety, and have poorer social skills and confidence would be more likely to use the Internet to escape from and avoid problems in real life, and this could lead to negative outcomes.

Studies present some interesting evidence on the association of personality characteristics and online relationship formation. The first HomeNet study was a longitudinal investigation of 93 non-representative families in the Pittsburgh area. They were provided with computers and an Internet connection free of charge for three years. The study found extroversion was negatively related to frequency of Internet use; introverts were more likely to be frequent Internet users (Kraut et al., 1998). Internet effects proved to differ according to personality characteristics, in particular, extroversion/introversion. The authors found support for "the rich get richer hypothesis": extroverts reported more Internet use and creating more online relationships. Introverts who used the Internet extensively reported less social involvement. In sum, Internet use was associated with better outcomes for extroverts and worse outcomes for introverts. In particular, extroverts who used the Internet more reported increased well-being, including low levels of loneliness. In contrast, introverts who were heavy Internet users showed a decline in their well-being (Kraut et al., 2002). The HomeNet study was based on the dystopian assumption (see Preface) that the Internet exerts negative effects on the individual's well-being, partly because of another assumption that time invested in the Internet is non-social time, diverted from other sources of sociability.

Others who subscribe to these perspectives have investigated the link between personal attributes and online activities, such as sensation-seeking and Internet dependence (Lin and Tsai, 2002). The social needs outlook has found much corroboration in social psychology. A study in Holland with a sample of 687 adolescents investigated personality characteristics and the perception of online communication. Socially anxious and lonely adolescents were found to value online communication more strongly. Youngsters with these personality characteristics perceived the Internet as providing them with more opportunities to reflect and control the messages they sent, and they perceived online communication as deeper and more reciprocal than face-to-face communication (Peter and Valkenburg, 2006). Similarly, in Germany, Wolfradt and Doll (2001) investigated the relation between extroversion/introversion and three Internet uses (information, entertainment, and interpersonal communication) among 122 adolescent Internet users. The social needs hypothesis was mainly supported by specific personality traits, such as neuroticism, which was proved to be positively associated with the entertainment motive and with the interpersonal communication motive; extroversion was positively associated with the communication motive only. Wolfradt and Doll (2001) argued accordingly that personality traits predict corresponding types of Internet activities. All in all, existing knowledge indicates that personality characteristics are influential in the use and choice of this medium for relationship formation. Online communication is an important means for socially anxious, introverted, and lonely adolescents to overcome their inhibitions in face-to-face settings. The Internet not only offers such young people a new venue to fulfill the need for association and involvement in a social circle, it also compensates for their lack of social skills and ultimately may help them to gain self-confidence, to be enjoyed later in face-to-face interactions.

The association between online communication and relational closeness is particularly interesting. Using a large sample of Dutch youth aged 12–17 years, Valkenburg and Peter (2007a) investigated whether online communication stimulated or reduced closeness to friends, and whether intimate disclosure of personal information online affected their closeness to online ties. These authors found that only 30 percent of the adolescents perceived online communication as effective in disclosing personal information. Furthermore, online communication with others whom they met online proved to have a negative effect on the perceived closeness to friends (Valkenburg and Peter, 2007a).

The social compensation hypothesis

On the contrary, the social compensation hypothesis proposes that individuals with higher levels of social anxiety or lower levels of social support, use social media to create online relationships to compensate for their lack of social ties, as social anxiety is a barrier for the creation of offline relationships (Van Ingen and Wright, 2016). According to this hypothesis, the relative anonymity of social media and the process of self-disclosure online provide individuals with a more comfortable social situation due to a perceived lower risk for self-disclosure because of the lack of nonverbal cues (Schouten et al., 2007). Furthermore, the Internet may provide more opportunities for some people to gain social support, explore their self-identities and social identities, and improve their social skills, as well as a greater opportunity to use online coping resources (Van Ingen and Wright, 2016). Additionally, Ellison et al. (2007) proposed that online activities were beneficial for individuals to form weak ties in social networking, which would be very useful for those with lower self-esteem to improve their social capital but would be harmful for those with higher self-esteem since it would reduce their opportunities to maintain their strong offline ties. In other words, "the poor get richer" and "the rich get poorer."

Social diversification

As discussed, most of the previous perspectives focus on personality characteristics as motivations for online relationship formation. The social diversification perspective relies on social network and social capital assumptions to explain variations in these motivation for disadvantaged groups in society.

The social diversification hypothesis deals specifically with differences in the use of communication and information technologies among racial and ethnic minorities (Mesch and Talmud, 2010; Gonzales, McCrory, Calarco, and Lynch, 2018). Relying on the literature demonstrating the stratification of multicultural societies along ethnic and social class lines, the social diversification hypothesis argues that network-based social closure affects the ability to obtain social capital and is more likely to benefit the dominant group's members (Mesch et al., 2012). According to this perspective, social media platforms might support the expansion of social relationships, including improving access to information, knowledge, and skills that are unavailable locally, and provide opportunities for the diversification of social relationships (Mesch and Talmud, 2010). As Mazur and Kozarian (2010) found in their study of older adolescents, despite the partial overlap of online and offline ties, online communication tends to diversify the structure of peer networks and expose youngsters to others who share their interests, regardless of their age, gender, or location. In that sense, the social diversification hypothesis argues that social media provides a platform for overcoming the existing segregation in society. Therefore, this perspective maintains that disadvantaged groups will have greater incentives to use Facebook to expand their social circle and overcome existing physical and social barriers to information and association. At the same time, majority groups will use the Internet to keep their existing relationships and maintain the closure of the network. In addition, they will be less likely than disadvantaged minorities to use Facebook to expand their social ties.

The social diversification perspective emphasizes the potential of social media platforms for empowering disadvantaged groups through affiliation with weak ties (Mazur and Kozarian, 2010). Indeed, a study of the online practices of young adolescents in a large rural area in California, planning for their vocational future, determined that the youngsters relied on computer-mediated communication and the establishment of contacts with weak ties to access information unavailable to them locally (Robinson, 2011). Similarly, the use of social media has been associated with the diversification of core networks of discussion (Hampton, Sessions, and Her, 2011). A study of a large sample of college students established that access to the Internet was still higher among White students than among Latinos and African Americans. However, when it comes to the use of social media platforms for content creation (blogs, video clips), a social capital-enhancing activity, Blacks and Hispanics reported a higher average of online content creation than Whites, even after controlling for socio-economic status, gender, and age, as well as Internet experience and psychological predictors (Correa and Jeong, 2011).

For young adolescents, SNSs may provide an opportunity to expand the size and composition of their social networks. Indeed, a study of

Internet use in a representative sample of Greek and Turkish youth in Cyprus suggests the existence of a reverse digital divide, as the more disadvantaged community engaged more often in Internet use for self-expression and association with weak ties (Milioni, Doudaki, and Demertzis, 2014). Mesch (2018a) conducted a test of this hypothesis and investigated the role of race and ethnicity in the self-reported strength of the social ties of young adolescents on Facebook. Based on the social diversification hypothesis, which argues that in multicultural societies, race and ethnicity are key factors that shape the nature of associations, we investigated whether there are ethnic and racial differences in the size and strength of the ties of adolescent Facebook users and the role of the strength of these ties in several positive outcomes. Using data from the US Teens' Social Media and Privacy Survey conducted by the Pew Research Center's Internet and American Life Project among 802 teens aged 12–17, we found no differences in the total number of ties that adolescents from different ethnic and racial groups reported. However, African Americans reported a significantly higher number of online weak ties, while White Americans had a significantly higher number of online strong ties. The results are consistent with the social diversification hypothesis.

Online ties and the structure of youth social networks

A prominent theme in the public discourse regarding social networks, reflected in the tone of many scholastic studies, is the claim that creating online social ties reduces the number of offline friends. Studies have warned that excessive Internet use may isolate adolescents from their friends. Available data indicate that the size of a social network is not affected by online relationship formation. A temporary decrease may be expected as more energy and time are invested in the creation of online ties; but over time, as online associations become integrated, the size of the network even slightly increases as new associations are added and old ones kept (Valkenburg and Peter, 2007b). In that sense, the effect of online relationship formation seems not to differ from the effect of cell phones. Igarashi, Takai, and Yoshida (2005), analyzing text messages over cell phones in Japan, found general support for the claim that mobile phones can change social networks among young people by increasing the number of possible contacts and promoting selective relationship formation. Mobile phones increase the frequency of communication, and allow opportunities for expanding interpersonal relationships.

The effect of expansion of social networks seem more pronounced on extroverts than on introverts, and varies according to attachment style, but overall, online relationship formation enlarges the social network for the majority of adolescents who choose to become involved in this activity (Mesch and Talmud, 2010).

Associating with similar people is another social network dimension influenced by online relationship formation. One of the most significant and consistent findings reported in the literature is that social relationships are characterized by social similarity, or homophily. Studies on the formation of close social relationships have emphasized the importance of social similarity in friendship and attraction in intimate social relationships. Similarity molds network ties, resulting in relatively homogeneous social networks in terms of socio-demographic, behavioral, and interpersonal characteristics. This tendency of individuals to associate with others who are similar to them has important social consequences. For example, similar individuals exchange information that suits their personal characteristics, preferences, and social style. Contacting similar individuals, however, limits personal social horizons, thus restricting the exposure to different others, thereby reproducing social stereotypes.

Studies found that adolescents who created online social ties also reported a higher heterogeneity of their social network by age, gender, and location. In an early study, Mesch and Talmud compared youngsters with online friends and with face-to-face friends for the respective average age difference between those friends and themselves (Mesch and Talmud, 2010). The former reported that their online friends were on average older than themselves; the latter did not report this. The difference was small, online friends being on average one year and a half older. Accordingly, to a certain extent, online friendship formation breaks through the barriers of age-grade segregation which is imposed by the social structure of schools.

An important dimension to consider is the perceived closeness of youth to their online ties, and its possible effect on their perceived closeness to their face-to-face ties. Online relationship formation is a dynamic process, and accordingly calls for longitudinal studies. The perception of being less close to online friends seems to depend on the developmental stage of the relationship. Online ties are relatively newer than face-to-face ties, and are based on narrower shared interests. Furthermore, it takes time to develop relationships. Hence, more investigation is required to examine the process of changing the perceived online ties' strength. Still, there is no evidence that youth are exchanging close offline friendships for distant and narrower ones. Online ties, then, do not seem to replace but to supplement face-to-face connections.

Studies comparing the percentage of friends of the opposite sex, as reported by youth with and without online friends, found less sex segregation for the former than for the latter (Mesch and Talmud, 2006a,

2006b). More to the point, adolescents whose friends were similar in age, ethnic background, and place of residence were more likely to report forming friendships online (Mesch and Talmud, 2006a, 2006b).

Another component of the shared opportunity for mutual exposure is residential proximity. Proximity facilitates the likelihood of friendship formation and communication by increasing the probability that individuals will meet and interact. Proximity is of particular importance for adolescents limited in their geographic mobility as they must rely on public transport, which is not always reliable. For adolescents who are restricted in their physical mobility, and for whom the main arenas of social interaction are the school, the neighborhood, and extracurricular activities, the Internet represents a new focus of common activities. Adolescents connect to the Internet, chat, and exchange emails with friends, with friends of friends, and with unknown individuals. In these activities they encounter a new space that facilitates joint activities and social interaction. For adults, as well as for a large majority of adolescents, the Internet is an innovative place for social interaction, different from the phone and television.

Quality of offline and online ties

One of the key features of friendships is their quality. The quality of friendships refers to the experienced closeness, trust, and understanding between friends. Several studies have investigated and compared the quality of online versus offline friendships (Mesch and Talmud, 2006a, 2006b). These studies have consistently demonstrated that online friendships are perceived to be lower in quality than offline friendships (Mesch and Talmud, 2006a). Furthermore, although the quality of both online and offline friendships increased over time, the quality of online friendships improved significantly more than offline relationships. Specifically, they discovered when online friendships lasted for more than a year, their quality became comparable to offline friendships.

The association between online communication and relational closeness is particularly interesting. Using a large sample of Dutch youth aged 12–17 years, Valkenburg and Peter (2007a) investigated whether online communication stimulated or reduced closeness to friends, and whether intimate disclosure of personal information online affected their closeness to online ties. These authors found that only 30 percent of the adolescents perceived online communication as effective in disclosing personal information. Furthermore, online communication with others whom they met online proved to have a negative effect on the perceived closeness to friends (Valkenburg and Peter, 2007a). A possible explanation for the perception of relational closeness of online ties is provided by an Israeli study with a large representative sample of adolescents, in which this perception was found to result from the length of communication. In fact, online ties are acquainted for less time than face-to-face ties, so they are still at the phase of relationship development and are therefore perceived to be of lesser depth and breadth (Mesch and Talmud, 2006b). Yet as time goes by, and as the topics of conversation expand from a small number of shared interests to a wider range, the perceived distance to online contacts is assumed to decrease.

Recent research

In the early days of ICT, the main distinction made was between online and offline ties. The definition of these ties was based on the origin of the relationship that often shaped the communication channels and the communication content. With the increase in Internet access, the proliferation of online platforms of communication (including social network sites, Instant Messaging, WhatsApp), the distinction became more difficult and today it is more reasonable to capture the social world of young and adults as being composed of online, offline, and mixed mode friendships. By mixed mode friendships, we mean the integration of online and offline ties and their interaction in our lives. Thus mixed mode friendships are the ones that originate online and extend to offline settings.

The notion of online relationship formation requires conceptual clarification. Most research has not clearly defined what is meant by online ties. It was largely conducted to elucidate the effects of channel characteristics on interpersonal communication, emphasizing the lack of social presence, lack of richness, and lack of clues in Internet communication and it sought the conditions under which this communication is non-personal or becomes hyper-personal (Walther, 1996). By contrast, in our view, the definition of online and face-to-face ties has to do more with the origin of the relationship and not with the mode of communication. This is a more pertinent perspective as social media has undergone significant convergence and has changed the domestication of ICT and youth sociability via digital social media (see Chapter 3). Youth communicate with close school friends using Instant Messaging, email, social networks sites, and school forums. In this case, someone can have friends whom one meets every day at school, yet conducts most of their communication online. Our interest lies mainly in the differences between online and face-to-face ties origination, so that our definition is that online ties refer to individuals who were first met online by means of applications, such as email, Instant Messaging, SNSs, chat rooms, or online game groups. According to our definition, then, a face-to-face friend is someone whom one met in person, in a setting such as school, the neighborhood, or other extracurricular activity (Mesch and Talmud, 2010).

How do online, offline, and mixed-mode friendships differ? Antheunis, Valkenburg and Peter (2012) conducted a study in which they compared the quality of online, offline, and mixed-mode friendships and the relative contribution of proximity, perceived similarity to the quality of friendship. The study was based on data gathered from a large sample of members of a Dutch social networking site (n = 2,188). An important finding is that differences in quality between online and offline friendships were found and remained significant over time, but those between mixed-mode and offline friendships disappeared. As already mentioned in the literature, the migration of a connection from being a person met online to one met face-to-face and voice-phone is an important step that increases the closeness between them. For that reason, mixed mode relationships tend to be more similar over time than solely face-to-face and only online ties.

The first question is the extent to which proximity and perceived similarity differ among online, mixed-mode, and offline friendships. The study found significant differences in the level of proximity between the types of friendship, the actual distance between offline friends is the lowest, followed by mixed-mode and online friends. As to perceived similarity between online, mixed-mode, and offline friendships. there is a significant difference in perceived similarity between the online and mixed-mode friendships, and between online and offline friendships. Perceived similarity was the highest in mixed-mode friendships and offline friendships, and lowest in online friendships (Antheunis et al., 2012).

In accordance with earlier studies, they found that respondents perceived offline friendships to be of higher quality than online friendships. However, the study also found that mixed-mode friendships, which are also formed online but then also migrate to offline communication modalities (i.e., telephone, face-to-face communication), were rated similar in quality as offline friendships. Thus, it is not important whether a friendship is formed online or offline, but rather, it is more important that newly formed friendships also migrate to cue-richer communication modalities, such as telephone and face-to-face contact friendships (Antheunis et al., 2012).

The study found that the quality of all three types of friendship improved as the friendship developed over time. The quality of online friendships remained significantly lower than that of offline friendships, even after two years. According to those authors:

- *Proximity.* They in fact found that offline friends lived closer to each other than mixed-mode and online friends. This suggests that in online and mixed-mode friendships, actual geographic proximity is less important to becoming friends.
- *Similarity.* they found that the level of perceived similarity was lower in online friendships compared to mixed-mode and offline friendships. They did find, however, that the effect of similarity on the quality of friendship was higher for online friendships than for mixed-mode and offline friendships. These results indicate that though the level of similarity is low in online friendships, similarity is a more important determinant of friendship quality in online friendships than in the other two categories of friendships (Antheunis et al., 2012).

Virtual interactions and online spaces are, in fact, additional sites of inter-action in which youth can explore their identities, belonging, and sense of themselves (Stern, 2004). As they get older, their Internet literacy as well as their tendency to share personal information seem to grow, though with limited understanding of the risks involved (Livingstone, 2008). Still, perceptions regarding the risk involved in online relations have been modified: while in 2003 distrust in online ties was associated with geo-graphical proximity between persons, the link between mistrust of the Internet to geographical proximity had disappeared between 2003 to 2006 (Dutton and Shepherd, 2003; Helsper, 2008b). Additionally, young people report a growing dependency on the Internet for activities ran-ging from managing their daily lives to building and maintaining online social interaction. The embeddedness of ICT in social structure creates a dual nature of communicative space, where both adolescents' offline and online domains serve as facilitators of communicative action in key life experiences (McMillan and Morrison, 2006). Over time, enthusiasm for meeting strangers on the Internet wanes, and reports of boredom surface, even among children (Livingstone and Bober, 2004).

In the context of the "fear of strangers," it is important to note the process of movement from online to face-to-face relationships. After the young people became acquainted online, and discovered common interests and topics of discussion, sometimes they would exchange emails, often using IM, then they communicate by phone, and finally in few cases they arranged to meet face-to-face in a public place. This is cautious progress, moving from online meeting as strangers, followed by a rise in the frequency of communication and in the number of its channels. The goal of these successive moves is the establishment of trust, resulting from progressive disclosure of personal information (Mesch and Talmud, 2007a).

Furthermore, the concept of the stranger is not always adequate to describe relationship formation online. Frequently, online communication and mobile communication are a way to introduce mutual friends to each other (Wolack et al., 2003). This happens when a new friend is introduced to an existing group or when an adolescent suggests to another friend that he or she meet a new person who has the same interests or the same personal problems.

Interpersonal lives and the computer and mobile activities of early adolescents reflexively amplify each other. Contemporary moral development is less about mastering distinctly right and wrong answers, and more about negotiating different social contexts. Additionally, even in a CMC environment, interpersonal and even intimate clues can be possible (Walther, 1996). There is evidence that the number of personal relationships occurring via the Internet is increasing as more people gain access to it (Underwood and Findlay, 2004; Lawson and Leck, 2006). What adolescents do after school hours, through the windows of their computer screens, has become an integral and important part of their individual and social identity formation and of their moral development (Bradley, 2005).

Valentine and Holloway (2002) found a rich variety of adolescents' strategies to reconfigure their personal activities between offline and online spaces. The study found four ways in which adolescents, aged 11–16, incorporated their offline worlds and their online spaces: (1) by direct (re)presentations of their offline identities and activities; (2) by the production of alternative identities also contingent on their offline identities; (3) by the reproduction online of offline class and gender divides; and (4) by reducing the ways in which everyday material realities limit the scope of their online activities. These authors also identified three different processes whereby adolescents incorporate online space into their offline worlds: (1) online activities maintain and develop both distant and local offline relationships; (2) information gathered online is incorporated into offline activities; and (3) online friendships are incorporated into or reconfigure offline social networks and position within networks (Valentine and Holloway, 2002).[1]

Notwithstanding important, adolescents' conduct offline seems similar to their conduct online. Their ways of social coping online and offline are markedly associated. Seepersad (2004) found a strong relationship between avoidant coping strategies offline and Internet use for entertainment. Moreover, adolescents who considered communication the most important use of the Internet also contended with loneliness through expression of emotion and social coping. Results suggest that online and offline coping behaviors are strongly related, especially if they are avoidant

(Seepersad, 2004). Many positive and negative developmental behaviors, such as dating, smoking, formation of musical tastes and frictional violence, are transferred via adolescents' peer social networks (Neal, 2007).

Adolescent friendships, networked individuals, and the information society

For some young users, the Internet is becoming another location to meet and socialize, and relations created there tend to migrate to other settings too (Wolak et al., 2003; Mesch and Levanon, 2003). As young people become less controlled by traditional social authorities, they can overstep their geographical limits and their local groups' boundaries, using electronic communication technologies (Wellman, 2001).

The Internet is typically used by adolescents as an additional space of activity and social interaction, which often complements rather than replaces offline spaces of social communication, activity, and gathering. Networked publics provide an additional virtual context for youth to develop social norms in negotiation with their peers, forming social ties, maintaining friendship networks, and accruing information and entertainment items and devices from remote environments. The adolescent is a sophisticated "networked individual," who negotiates a wider range of messages and identities using multiple means of computer-mediated, mobile, and face-to-face channels of communication.

Adolescents' online activity and subculture are unique. This distinctiveness stems from both an age effect and a generational effect. The age effect refers to the influence of life-stage characteristics on adolescents' social conduct and network structure. The generational (or cohort) effect refers to the cultural change adolescents are exposed to in their formative years. Nowadays computer and Internet literacy, online communication, smartphone and hyper-textual literacy are skillfully mastered. Social networks sites are unique artefacts that allow early adolescents to share and discuss ideas and feelings, ask and answer each other's questions, or showcase projects, all of which promote a pro-social attitude. If in the past the formation of the youth culture was limited to neighborhood hangouts, now spaces and channels of interaction are expanded, allowing individuals to find peers to share interests, hobbies, and feelings conditional upon having access and skills.

Expansion of weak ties via online social networks compensates, in particular, youth with deprived life outcomes. A study of social networks sites has suggested a close association between the use of Facebook and social capital, the firmest relationship being with "bridging" social capital. In addition, Facebook usage was found to interact with measures of psychological well-being, suggesting that it might provide greater benefits for users experiencing low self-esteem and low life satisfaction (Ellison, Steinfield, and Lampe, 2007).

Typically, adolescents' offline networks are denser and much more age- and sex-homogeneous than those of adults. Typically, adults also have more options to form new social ties, drawn from more diversified social foci of activity, than adolescents. Peer-group pressure on adolescents is more likely to encourage dense social ties, comprising of closely knit, transitive relations (in which a person's friends know his or her third parties as well), which tend to be geographically proximate as well.

In our view, the digital communication space reflects the social structure, its access and use are dependent on the social stratification process. Individuals bring to their online participation the diverse social status that they occupy and their social norms of behavior. Yet, at the same time online communication exerts some transformative effects on adolescents' behavior and friendship formation. Conceptualizing the Internet as foci of activity, we argue that technology is embedded in social structure. Digital platforms are another sphere of social interaction and action, where social agents play digital games, and exchange information, give and gain social support, and other instrumental and expressive resources. Thus, digital platforms are conceived as a social arena of shared and integrated activities. Hence, the social context molds relationship formation, not merely individual motivations and preferences. Technological features impact the use of digital platforms as well, by reducing costs, proximity considerations, and scope of choice among various channels of synchronous and asynchronous communication devices. Digital social interaction embeds certain properties from adolescents' offline social networks as well as from the digital environment; these act as social contextual facilitators, relevant to online sociability. These properties are in fact social affordance devices, bringing individuals together for purposes that create opportunities for social interaction, and introducing individuals to one another.

A comprehensive survey of 1,303 adolescents in Seoul, Singapore, and Taipei found that the Internet users among them differed in their Internet connectedness patterns in the nature of their social environments, in their family social status, and in other environmental factors (Jung, Lin, and Cheong, 2005). Most notably, the rate of Internet adoption by peers was an important factor explaining social media use. As the proportion of friends using the Internet increased, the more likely was the user to find technical support and to broaden and intensify online communication, thus increasing the likelihood of connecting through digital spaces. Considering that online activities are more likely to be shared among peers, the high rate of participation in these activities suggests a strong effect of peer groups in the likelihood of conducting communication is digital spaces (Jung, Lin and Cheong, 2005).

Effects of online relationship formation on social networks

The last part of this chapter is dedicated to understanding some of the potential effects of online relationship formation on young people's social circle. Table 4.1 presents the different perspectives on online relationship formation.

An important dimension of social networks, and one at the center of many studies, is the extent that its use reduces, enlarges, or does not change the number of friends. Studies have warned that excessive use of digital spaces may isolate adolescents from their friends. As we saw in Chapter 3, the available data indicate that the size of a social network is not negatively affected by online relationship formation. A temporary decrease may be expected as more energy and time are invested in

Table 4.1 Perspectives on online relationship formation

Disciplinary origin	Perspective	Implications
Psychology	Motivation theory	Correlation between personality traits and communication needs and gratification
	Social needs	Either the expansion of social ties, or the compensation for face-to-face relationship scarcity
	Sensation seeking Intimacy theory	Compensation for anxiety, isolation, or stimuli
Social structural	Dual embeddedness	Reconfiguration of communication strategies; coping in virtual space is similar to offline life
	Social affordance	Information spreads rapidly in CMC, but neither universally nor homogeneously
	Social network analysis	Homophily and transitivity drive relationship formation, but online relations are larger in size, weaker, and more sparse

the creation of online ties; but over time, as online associations become integrated, the size of the network even slightly increases as new associations are added and old ones kept (Mesch and Talmud, 2006a; Valkenburg and Peter, 2007b). In that sense, the effect of online relationship formation seems not to differ from the effect of cell phones. Igarashi, Takai, and Yoshida (2005), analyzing text messages over cellular phones in Japan, found general support for the claim that mobile phones can change social networks among young people by increasing the number of possible contacts and promoting selective relationship formation. Mobile phones increase the frequency of communication, and allow opportunities for expanding interpersonal relationships.

The effect of expansion of social networks seem more pronounced on extroverts than on introverts, and varies according to attachment style, but, overall, online relationship formation enlarges the social network for the majority of adolescents who choose to become involved in this activity (Buote et al., 2009; Hamburger and Ben-Artzi, 2000).

Associating with similar people is another social network dimension influenced by online relationship formation. One of the most significant and consistent findings reported in the literature is that social relationships are characterized by social similarity, or homophily. Studies on the formation of close social relationships have emphasized the importance of social similarity in friendship and attraction in intimate social relationships. Similarity molds network ties and results in homogeneous social networks in terms of socio-demographic, behavioral, and interpersonal characteristics. This tendency of individuals to associate with others who are similar to them has important social consequences. For example, similar individuals exchange information that suits their personal characteristics and social style. By mutual influence or by association, they reject social links and information coming from others who differ from them in social attributes, attitudes, or values. Contact with similar individuals limits one's personal social horizons, restricting exposure to different others, thereby reproducing social stereotypes.

Perceiving oneself as being less close to online friends seems to depend on the developmental stage of the relationship. Online ties are relatively newer than face-to-face ties, and are based on narrow shared interests. Relationships take time to develop and the process of moving from being perceived as less close requires more investigation. Regarding their effect on existing ties, there is no evidence that youth are exchanging close friendships for distant and narrow ones. Online ties, then, seem not to replace but to supplement face-to-face connections.

A highly consistent finding in the literature is that school years are characterized by gender-based segregation. There is evidence that the extent of segregation decreases over the years, in particular from middle school to high school, but it remains relatively high even at the end of high school (Shrum, Cheek, and Hunter, 1988). Studies have shown that in adolescence there is a "sex cleavage" in friendship relations (Cotterell, 1996). In our study, we compared the percentage of friends of the opposite sex as reported by youth with and without online friends. We found less sex segregation for the former than for the latter (Mesch and Talmud, 2006a). Adolescents whose friends were similar in age, ethnic background, and place of residence were more likely to report forming friendships online (Mesch and Talmud, 2006a).

Summary

In this chapter we have discussed how online spaces are used in the context of relationship formation and the creation of friendship ties by means of ICT. We have emphasized the role of online communication as providing an alternative and also a complementary space for relationship formation, given the specific restrictions that youth face. These constraints are mainly geographic, constituting a contextual barrier that motivates some adolescents to turn to the Internet in seeking others who share their specific interests or differ in their racial/ethnic background and social characteristics. Heterogeneity in adolescents' social networks, occurring more often when the origin of the friendship is online, has developmental implications that require further investigation. For example, Stanton-Salazar and Spina (2005) found that non-romantic, cross-gender online relationships between adolescents proved an important source of social support. They afforded emotional support, particularly for the males. If the Internet reduces friendship gender segregation for young adolescents, this in the future may have an impact on the process of dating and first-time sexual relationships. Another potential effect is in the early exposure to individuals of diverse ethnic and racial groups and of varying political views. If this is confirmed in future research, digital spaces are very likely to become a central agent of socialization, which has to be integrated into our understanding of youth socialization.

The existing division in research between the "virtual" and the "real" does not of course accurately capture the lived social experiences and identity negotiations of adolescents in their socialization process, nor their belonging to peer groups, nor does it encompass the complexity in which offline and online spaces are mutually embedded.

The emergence of ICT into adolescents' identity management, personal communities, and friendship formation seems to have changed the character of "private" and "public" spaces, constituted by adolescents' activities on and around the screen. In Chapter 5, we connect elements of offline and online interactions regarding the maintenance and expansion of social ties, and the diversification of social networks through ICT.

Note

1 For a general theory considering the reconfiguration of ICT communication, see Walther (1996).

Bibliography

Antheunis, M.L., Valkenburg, P.M., and Peter, J. (2012) The quality of online, offline, and mixed-mode friendships among users of a social networking site, *Cyberpsychology: Journal of Psychosocial Research on Cyberspace*, 6(3), Article 6. https://doi.org/10.5817/CP2012-3-6.

Boase, J. and Wellman, B. (2006) Personal relationships: on and off the internet, in D. Perlman and A.L. Vangelistihe (Eds.), *Handbook of Personal Relations*, Cambridge: Cambridge University Press.

Bradley, K. (2005) Internet lives: social context and moral domain in adolescent development, *New Directions for Youth Development*, 108, 57–76.

Buote, V.M., Wood, E. and Pratt, M. (2009) Exploring similarities and differences between online and offline friendships: the role of attachment style, *Computers in Human Behavior*, 25, 560–567.

Chen, W., Boase, J., and Wellman, B. (2002) The global villagers, in B. Wellman and C. Haythornthwaite (Eds.), *The Internet in Everyday Life*, Oxford: Blackwell, pp. 74–113.

Cohen, A.A., Lamish, D., and Schejter, A.M. (2008) The wonder phone in the land of miracles: mobile telephony in Israel, *New Media: Policy and Social Research Issues*, Cresskill, NJ: Hampton Press.

Correa, T. and Jeong, S.H. (2011) Race and online content creation: why minorities are actively participating in the Web, *Information, Communication and Society*, 14(5), 638–659.

Cotterell, J. (1996) *Social Networks and Social Influences in Adolescence*, London: Routledge.

Dutton, W.H. and Shepherd, A. (2003) Trust in the Internet: the social dynamics of an experience technology. Research Report No. 3, Oxford: Oxford Internet Institute.

Ellison, N.B., Steinfeld, C., and Lampe, C. (2007) The benefits of Facebook "friends:" social capital and college students' use of online social network sites, *Journal of Computer Mediated Communication*, 12, 1143–1168.

Gonzales, A., McCrory Calarco, J., and Lynch, T. (2018) Technology problems and student achievement gaps: a validation and extension of the technology maintenance construct, *Communication Research*. https://doi.org/10.1177/0093650218796366.

Hamburger, Y.A. and Ben-Artzi, E. (2000) The relationship between extraversion and neuroticism and the different uses of the Internet, *Computers in Human Behavior*, 16, 441–449.

Hampton, K.N., Sessions, L.F., Her, E.J., and Rainie, L. 2009. *Social Isolation and New Technology*, Washington, DC: Pew Internet and American Life Project.

Hampton, K.N. and Wellman, B. (2002) The not so global village of Netville, in B. Wellman and C. Haythornthwaite (Eds.), *The Internet in Everyday Life*, Oxford: Blackwell, pp. 345–372.

Helsper, E.J. (2008a) Gendered internet use across generations and life stages in the UK. Paper presented at AOIR Conference, Copenhagen, October.

Helsper, E.J. (2008b) Perceptions of security and risks on the internet: experience and learned levels of trust. Presentation slides from IT Security in Practice Conference, Aarhus University, January 24.

Igarashi, T., Takai, J., and Yoshida, T. (2005) Gender differences in social network development via mobile phone text messages: a longitudinal study, *Journal of Social and Personal Relationships*, 22(5), 691–713.

Jung, J.Y., Kim, Y.C., Lin, W.Y., and Cheong, P.H. (2005) The influence of social environment on internet, connectedness of adolescents in Seoul, Singapore and Taipei, *New Media and Society*, 7(1), 64–88.

Kadushin, C. (2004) *Understanding Social Networks: Theories, Concepts, and Findings*. Oxford: Oxford University Press.

Khan, S., Gagné, M., Yang, L., and Shapka, J. (2016) Exploring the relationship between adolescents' self-concept and their offline and online social worlds, *Computers in Human Behavior*, 55, 940–945.

Kraut, R., Kiesler, S., Boneva, B., Cummings, J., Helgeson, V., and Crawford, A. (2002) Internet paradox revisited, *Journal of Social Issues*, 58, 49–74. https://doi.org/10.1111/1540-4560.00248.

Kraut, R., Patterson, M., Lundmark, V., Kiesler, S., Mukopadhyay, T., and Scherlis, W. (1998) Internet paradox: a social technology that reduces social involvement and psychological well-being?, *American Psychologist*, 53, 1011–1031.

Lawson, H. and Leck, K. (2006) Dynamics of internet dating, *Social Science Computer Review*, 24(2), 189–208.

Lenhart, A. (2009) It's personal: similarities and differences in online social network use between teens and adults. Available at: www.pewinternet.org/Presentations/2009/19-Similarities-and-Differences-in-Online-Social-Network-Use.aspx.

Lin, S.S.J. and Tsai, C.C. (2002) Sensation seeking and internet dependence of Taiwanese high school adolescents, *Computers in Human Behavior*, 18(4), 411–426.

Livingstone, S. (2008) Taking risky opportunities in youthful content creation: teenagers' use of social networking sites for intimacy, privacy and self expression, *New Media and Society*, 10(3), 393–411.

Livingstone, S. and Bober, M. (2004) *U.K. Children Go Online*, London: London School of Economics.

Mazur, E. and Kozarian, L. (2010) Self-presentation and interaction in blogs of adolescents and young emerging adults, *Journal of Adolescent Research*, 25(1), 124–144. https://doi.org/10.1177/0743558409350498.

McMillan, S.J. and Morrison, M. (2006) Coming of age with the internet: a qualitative exploration of how the internet has become an integral part of young people's lives, *New Media and Society*, 8(1), 73–95.

Mesch G.S. (2018a) Race, ethnicity and the strength of Facebook ties, *Journal of Youth Studies* 21(5), 575–589.

Mesch, G.S. and Levanon, Y. (2003) Community networking and locally based social ties in two suburban localities, *City and Community*, 2, 335–351.

Mesch G.S. and Talmud, I. (2006a) Online friendship formation, communication channels, and social closeness, *International Journal of Internet Sciences*, 1(1), 29–44.

Mesch, G.S. and Talmud, I. (2006b) The quality of online and offline relationships, the role of multiplexity and duration, *The Information Society*, 22(3), 137–148.

Mesch, G.S. and Talmud, I. (2007a) Similarity and the quality of online and offline social relationships among adolescents in Israel, *Journal of Research in Adolescence*, 17(2), 455–465.

Mesch, G.S. and Talmud, I. (2010) Internet connectivity, community participation, and place attachment: a longitudinal study, *American Behavioral Scientist*, 53(8), 1095–1110.

Mesch, G.S. Quase-Han, A., and Talmud, I. (2012) IM social networks: individual, relational and cultural characteristics, *Journal of Personal and Social Relationships*, 29(6), 736–759.

Milioni, D.L., Doudaki, V., and Demertzis, N. (2014) Youth, ethnicity, and a 'reverse digital divide': a study of internet use in a divided country, *Convergence*, 20, 316–336.

Neal, J.W. (2007) Why social networks matter: a structural approach to the study of relational aggression in middle childhood and adolescence, *Child and Youth Care Forum*, 36, 195–211.

Peter, J. and Valkenburg, P.M. (2006) Research note: individual differences in perception of internet communication, *European Journal of Communication*, 21(2), 213–226.

Robinson, L. (2011) Information-channel preferences and information-opportunity structures, *Information, Communication and Society*, 14(4), 472–494.

Shrum, W., Cheek Jr, N.H., and Hunter S. (1988) Friendship in school: gender and racial homophily, *Sociology of Education*, 61, 227–239.

Sproull, L. and Kiesler, S. (1986) Reducing social context cues: electronic email in organizational communications, *Management Science*, 32, 1492–1512.

Stanton-Salazar, R.D. and Spina, S.U. (2005) Adolescent peer networks as a context for social and emotional support, *Youth and Society*, 36(4), 379–417.

Stern, S.R. (2004) Expressions of identity online: prominent features and gender differences in adolescents' world wide web home pages, *Journal of Broadcasting and Electronic Media*, 48(2), 218–243.

Underwood, H. and Findlay, B. (2004) Internet relationships and their impact on primary relationships, *Behaviour Change*, 21(2), 127–140.

Valentine, G. and Holloway, S.L. (2002) Cyberkids? Exploring children's identities and social networks in on-line and off-line worlds, *Annals of the Association of American Geographers*, 92(2), 302–319.

Valkenburg, P.M. and Peter, J. (2007a) Preadolescents' and adolescents' online communication and their closeness to friends, *Developmental Psychology*, 43(2), 267–277.

Valkenburg, P.M. and Peter, J. (2007b) Online communication and adolescent wellbeing: testing the stimulation versus the displacement hypothesis, *Journal of Computer-Mediated Communication*, 12, 1169–1182.

Van Ingen, E., and Wright, K.B. (2016) Predictors of mobilizing online coping versus offline coping resources after negative life events, *Computers in Human Behavior*, 59, 431–439.

Walther, J.B. (1996) Computer-mediated communication: impersonal, interpersonal and hyperpersonal interaction, *Communication Research,* 23(1), 3–43.

Wellman, B. (2001) Computer networks as social networks, *Science*, 293, 2031–2034.

Wolak, J., Mitchell, K.J., and Finkelhor, D. (2003) Escaping or connecting? Characteristics of youth who form close online relationships, *Journal of Adolescence*, 26, 105–119.

Wolfradt, U. and Doll, J. (2001) Motives of adolescents to use the internet as a function of personality traits, personal and social factors, *Educational Computing Research*, 24(1), 13–27.

8

IDENTITY CITIZENSHIP

Authenticity, intersectionality and a new populism

Rob Cover

Introduction: the cultural production of a new taxonomy online

Over the past chapters I have been presenting and analysing the recent emergence of a new taxonomy of gender and sexuality comprised of new identity labels, developments in the range of attraction types (beyond romantic and sexual), and new languages for addressing and representing gender (cisgender, transgender and non-binary gender). These have significant implications for contemporary culture in that they challenge the dominant understandings of identity that have remained relatively stable across the twentieth and early twenty-first centuries. An important point that I have referred to several times is the fact that these new ways of thinking about sexuality, gender and relationships first appear in online settings, principally social networking sites that have become popular places for discussing social justice causes, such as Tumblr, as well as dating sites and in more 'mainstream' online practices such as the use of Facebook. These have been significant in facilitating the kinds of conversations that can bring to light a new discursive arrangement – the networking of the excluded, the disenfranchised and the marginalised can make new identities possible, and these identities can be constituted in a sense of virtual community that sees itself as oppositional to the dominant or empowered.

While digital media has thus afforded the production of a broad new taxonomy of (continuously proliferating) labels, categories and classifications of sexuality and gender, it is likewise not necessarily helpful to understand digital media as the *source* or *cause* of this emergence. Rather, it is important to ask instead what might be the cultural conditions that prompt the contemporary emergence of new sexual subjectivities, since these arise by neither accident nor deliberate design but, as with all cultural shifts, through positionings and tensions between historical continuities and ruptures. In that context, I would like to begin this chapter by giving an overview of the specific role of digital media in affording the emergence of the new taxonomy of gender/sexual subjecthood through its capacity to foster and host interactivity, identity performativity online, and networked facilitation of political engagement. In showing that digital media facilitates the setting for emergence but does not cause it, I would like to use this chapter to discuss five factors which may be considered to be among the cultural structures, norms, disciplinary and biopolitical circumstances that foster the development of the new taxonomy.

These five factors are as follows: (1) the framework of *sexual citizenship* as a way of making sense of sexual and gender identities; (2) what I refer to as the *cult of authenticity* that demands subjects are answerable always 'as subjects', whereby categories – no matter how many or how proliferate – are the most efficient mechanism by which to measure the legitimacy of subjecthood; (3) the *demands of inclusivity* which provide an impetus for ensuring that subjects can find a grounding in a categorised gender and sexuality; (4) the *anti-fluidity backlash* that, in several ways, has sponsored the cultural desire or demand for more discrete, sensible and organised classifications of identity upon which diverse behaviours, desires, attractions and experiences can be mapped; and, finally (5) the role of *populism* as a particular cultural practice of anti-institutionalism and anti-expertise, differing somewhat from earlier decades of avant-garde artistic, political and liberatory practice. Together, these five cultural phenomena are implicated in the conditions that shape the need, desire or demand for an alternative framework of sexuality and gender identity. I will discuss each of these after pointing to some of the ways in which digital media enables them to produce forms of contemporary emergence.

The affordances of digital identity for a new taxonomy

Digital interactivity, and the co-creativity it proscribes, has been one of the most powerful settings making possible emergent re-conceptualisations of language, identity, subjectivity, gender and sexuality. Digital media, as I have previously argued, operate as a most efficient and most effective tool for individual and community identity construction, performance, recognition, reflection and self-articulation (Cover 2016). Helen Kennedy (2006) pointed out more than a decade ago that webpages, which are one among many forms of digital communication, are a media type marked by being never entirely quite finished, just as identity composition itself is a continuous process: both are constantly "under construction" (p. 869). In the same way, more recent, interactive forms of digital community-focused and network-building communication such as social networking pages, YouTube content, commentary and responses across forums and image-hosting databases and so on are the sites at which identity becomes most pointed and notable. This partly results from the debates around identity authenticity operating in those spaces, but also party because the sites themselves are geared to encourage a particular kind of identitarian reflectiveness as a central part of their process (Cover 2014). Unlike both face-to-face communication and early Web 1.0 communication, interactive social networking has encouraged the practice of articulating self-labels for sexual and gender identity in ways which have helped challenge the strictures of more simplistic binary-based hetero/homo-sexualities and masculine/feminine exclusive genders.

To put this another way, contemporary digital media culture enables the *intelligibility* of the cultural practices of gender and sexuality identity formation to be channelled differently via a range of mechanisms that relate to the *relationship between communication, form, engagement and – especially – identity as constituted in discourse*. It is helpful to think through the ways in which new practices emerge as a result of new ways of thinking that are produced through digital, networked engagement, that which Daniel Miller and Jolynna Sinanan (2014) have referred to as 'attainment'. Attainment here accepts and understands digital technologies as aspects of human relationality rather than as objects that detract from or disrupt our humanity. In that context, digital media does not produce a set of sexual and gender identity categories that are 'alien' to extant cultural practices but prompts the production of both continuities and change.

So, what are the digital mechanisms that enable the production of new taxonomies of gender and sexuality? To think about this involves unpacking some of the different aspects and elements of digital media itself, for it is not and never has been just one practice, artefact, or experience. There are four that are important to consider: (1) the fact that digital media is a site for the conveyance of discourse that permits us to encounter new information, resources, categories, labels and ways of thinking that may have previously been unavailable in our lives; (2) the way in which interactivity involves opportunities not just for encountering and reading identity discourses but asks us to participate and engage with them as co-creative participants; (3) the uses of social networking for identity performativity that complexify subjecthood but ask us to think about our selfhood, including gender and sexuality, in ways which replicate 'conversational' and self-reflective engagement; and, lastly (4) the affordances of digital media in bringing together a range of different voices, including the voices of the marginalised and disenfranchised that, together, enable the challenging of norms and the sharing of new, alternative frameworks for discussing gender and sexual subjectivity. Digital media culture and digital technologies operate both as sites for *representing* identity (categories, selves) and sites for *performing* our identity (articulations, play, engagement, images and so on), and it is therefore important to delineate some of these different aspects rather than assume that all online engagement is the same, or that the Internet is a singular concept, activity and formation.

Firstly, we have the fact that digital media is a site for providing vast quantities of information – the discourses which make intelligible the cultural demands of gender and sexuality coherence. It is not simply that they are *there* and that there is a range to choose from, but that there is an interpellative effect in the 'encounter' with those discourses which can inaugurate us to commence a new kind of gender or sexual performativity, including perhaps one which we did not think possible. For example, the information on heteroflexibility as an identity label, or non-binary as a gender label, might be encountered in an online setting – indeed the most likely place to find these terms at present. In encountering, we may find enough of a 'fit' with how we perceive ourselves or might find that our questions about sexual or gender coherence in ourselves are answered by those labels. The outcome is, in the right circumstances and with the right conditions, that we go on to cite the label and the behavioural information that goes along with it, to re-configure or reconstitute our sense of selfhood and to stabilise and sustain such performances over time in both our online and offline engagement.

Key to making sense of this is the figuration of 'encounter'. Neither digital media, nor the technological use of it, nor the information, resources or discourses encountered on it *determine* who and what we are. Important here is that in thinking about the role of digital media we don't think of it in a 'media effects' capacity (McKee 2012, p. 505), which would be to understand the content of what we find online and the interactive activities of engaging with it as determining and causing our gender and sexual identities, and new configurations of it, in the act of reading or seeing it online. Such effects models, including those which, for example, assume gaming will cause violent behaviours, online pornography will cause sexual assault or right-wing propaganda will produce neo-Nazis, underestimate the complex practices of reading, interpreting, critiquing and self-reflecting that are a very significant part of the media audience process. Important, then, is recognising that while we might first *encounter* some of the new discourses, categories and labels in online settings, those same settings are also places and instances of identity *performance*. In her book *Bodies That Matter* (1993), Judith Butler went to considerable lengths to demonstrate that while identity might be a performance, it is never in itself a voluntary, conscious or deliberate individual act. Rather, it is "always a reiteration of a norm or set of norms" (p. 12). That is, a subject does not express or articulate an inner truth, but cites, repeats and mimes the norms, attributes and codes of coherent behaviour that *fabricate* the idea there is an inner essence (Butler 1990, p. 136).

We encounter the 'norms' of gender and sexuality in a range of settings – gender in particular from the very first days of life, with a number of disciplinary practices at play to ensure coherent gender performances as either masculine or feminine and some safeguards to ensure that there is limited confusion, mixing up, play or transition. Sexuality and sexual information has traditionally been made available a little later, typically less available to the very young. This implies that in the case of sexuality, there is always an encounter with the discourses that make the sexual meaningful. Such encounters may be through film and television content (Cover 2000), formal and informal sex education (Rasmussen 2006), news stories and even graffiti (Leap 1996). Today, it is very clear that digital media is providing sexual informational resources and entertainment most actively. The encounter with discourses of sexuality that provide the 'resource' of coherent performances through categories, names, classifications, expected behaviours, intelligibilities and coherences are meaningful and significant for the constitution of sexual subjecthood. It is in the moment of encounter with, say, the dominant discourse of sexuality as a binary-based, fixed and essential division into hetero/homo that a process of recognisable sexual subjectivity is inaugurated and a trajectory for a 'lesbian' or 'gay' or 'straight' subjectivity is initiated.

In digital media terms, then, we see a certain set of differences from the dominant kinds of 'encounter' I am describing here. The practices through which gender and sexual identity are performative involve encountering the discourses and, in so doing, *citing* the name, category or signifier of sexual and gender subjectivity. In performing an identity – which is never a conscious or voluntary act – one thus cites and repeats the category and the information given culturally that makes that category intelligible and recognisable to oneself and to others. Such performances are repetitive and come to stabilise over time, retroactively producing the *illusion* that the performances manifest from a fixed, inner identity core (Butler 1990, p. 143). This continues, no matter how gender and sexuality might be figured. What I am arguing here, however, is that the category, name, norm and signifier are not only without fixity and foundation (Butler 1990, p. 147), but that in the context of digital media environments, they have shifted unexpectedly and substantially. So, for many younger persons and older persons as well, there is a new competing framework or language or taxonomy of gender (beyond masculine/feminine norms) and sexuality (beyond hetero/homo, bisexual and LGBT norms) made available in online settings that might differ from the expectations of gender and sexual identity norms recognisable in everyday dominant liberal–humanist frameworks.

Secondly, we have the *fact* of digital interactivity. In a traditional media and communication setting, the discourses that provide us with the information to make sense of gender categories and sexual identity categories have typically been provided to us through linear pathways of sender–message–receiver. That is, expert senders, and ourselves as involuntary receivers of the information and resources that tell us what a coherent and intelligible and acceptable gender or sexual identity is. These include the resources that also allow us to participate in our own disciplining, normalisation and self-policing of our performances. Interactivity is an everyday part of online engagement, and it very often involves processes of *making identification* or *articulating the self*. Pull-down menus that ask a subject to choose, for example, between two terms in a dichotomy open the possibility of thinking about that which is outside of the list (outside the frame), including what other possible ways there might be for defining ourselves (Griffin 2016, p. 148). So, for example, when a gender choice list only provides 'male' and 'female', we are tacitly invited to consider what kinds of alternatives there might be to those two terms. Of course, that does not mean that we do so in practice; however, the interactive setting of digital media in which some of our time is spent writing and some of our time spent clicking and choosing does open up those sorts of questions in a way the traditional paper form does not. The limitations of a menu and interactive call to utilise that menu when, for example, setting up a social networking profile, are thus put quite literally in front of our faces, hailing us not only to answer according to that dichotomy but also to 'answer back' by considering such lists' limitations.

At the same time, quizzes and online surveys on, for example, sexuality appear regularly online, including those which, as Donna Drucker (2012) has pointed to, utilise the Kinsey 0–6 scale, attempting to peg users' sexual identity according to six categories (numeric) rather than two (hetero/homo) or three (hetero/homo/bi), again requiring click-based responses to narrow available choices to describe sexual experience, desire and self-perception. This is, of course, a bastardised version of Kinsey that oversimplifies the framework (and a long way off from the Kinsey research team in-depth interviews); it relies more on categorisation against one of the six specific positions on the scale than on conceptualising sexuality along Kinsey's continuum. It is a good example of some of the ways in which digital media helps facilitate processes of categorisation and classification, particularly in the context of 'weak' kinds of interactivity (clicking) versus the more engaged, critical and nuanced practices of interactivity (writing, editing, remixing), a difference which is often forgotten in the marketing of the term interactivity (Cover 2006).

When we start thinking, however, about how interactivity occurs as a practice of textual engagement, we have to consider the central factor of *co-creativity* that encourages users to play with, shift and change texts. This is a practice, then, which has disrupted the normative way in which the 'encounter' with discourse has previously operated along linear terms of author–text–readership. Media, expertise, education and other discourses once dominated the provision of information resources which were encountered and served as the discursive source for gender and identity. The discourse, then, has been that which is constitutive, as it has been accessed, encountered, read and interpreted in an unassuming way. Now, in an interactive digital setting, what changes is that the discourse is no longer simply *given* and *encountered* in a linear sender–message–receiver model. Rather, it is open to the long-standing cultural demand that we participate in the stories that make our lives sensible (Cover 2006). That is, the participatory nature of contemporary digital media was not a new 'invention' that drastically changed how we communicate but can be understood as the fruition of some deeply held desires, cultural demands and attachments to participating in and sharing processes of authorship and creativity.

If identity is a citation of the identity that precedes and exceeds our selves in discourse (Butler 1993, pp. 225–226), and if that discourse is made available today primarily through forms of mediation, then in an increasingly online world in which user–participants are also active co-creators, the citation of a category, signifier, name or intelligibility is not only *conditioned* by communication technologies but is one to which we contribute *actively* and *creatively*. So, we now have to account not only for audience interpretation or activation of meanings in reception of discourses of gender and sexuality but also – today – for the interactive environment in which participation in the creation of the text itself becomes normative. Here, identity is produced simultaneously with interactive and co-creative production of the very discourses that are cited. We can see this best perhaps, for example, in the proliferate online practices of remixed texts such as audio-visual fan music videos, slash video, mash-ups and digital stories utilising and combining both existing and new visual and audio material on sites such as YouTube. Remixed texts are a new and transformative form of user engagement with media that makes use of older texts as 'found material' in order to produce an ostensibly intertextual experience (Lessig 2008, pp. 11–12); remix delivers forms of collage, complexity and co-creativity directed towards a broader audience. YouTube, for example, as a digital form encourages remix and consumer co-creation (Burgess and Green 2009, pp. 4–5) in a way which can upset, adjust, co-create or re-create the discourses of sexuality, gender, relationships and normativity.

A user might, say, take a number of scenes from a television series communicating gender and sexual norms in one way, re-sequence them into a new order, juxtaposed and aligned, and place them against an audio track sourced from somewhere completely differently. While independently the two sources might be reiterating and reinforcing dominant gender norms, the new remix content actively and creatively might produce a different kind of resource describing a more complex way of thinking about gender identity. This has been an outcome in much older slash video production, which has been part of audio and video remixing since the use in the 1970s of video recorders among television fans to create new gender and sexual meanings (Penley 1997). This practice adjusts representations of straight television characters by re-sequencing scenes, taking out-of-context clips, adding them to a meaningful song, all in order to 'queer' the characters and make them appear to be in a romantic same-sex relationship (Cover 2010). It might, too, be a product that achieves this unwittingly but allows new meanings to emerge. Within the framework of the new taxonomy of labels, however, we could also interactively 'queer' the discourse by remixing and sharing a series of texts that reproduces such characters as asexual, as non-binary or as any among the dozens and dozens of new identity labels. We could unwittingly complexify a romantic relationship to appear a 'platonic attraction' per the new typology of attractions discussed in Chapter 3. And in the act of doing this, we could find ourselves unwittingly critiquing a set of gender or sexual norms and producing new configurations that do not fit easily within the prevailing logic. In other words, an encounter with the discourse in an interactive, co-creative sense means precisely that we are co-creating the very discourses that give intelligibility to gender and sexuality in ways usually without intent.

This is not, then, simply the *productive activation* of meaning in the act of reading and interpreting a text, but the *active production* of new textualities produced in everyday practices of 'playing' with content that were previously unavailable or difficult to achieve prior to contemporary digital affordances. The extent to which such a new text might come to have new meanings for identity, creating new, unexpected and unanticipated categories, significations and attributes in which the reader recognises (and thereby is actively reconstituted as a new kind of self), will vary. Re-constitutive transformations of identity are theorised within Butler's work on performativity from the perspective of the encounter with new discourses that may have been previously unavailable to the subject (Butler 1991). In the context of digital interactivity as an everyday practice – including, particularly, those practices of digital engagement that are less-ostensibly 'creative' or 'artistic' – new discourses are produced by the subject, allowing wholly new configurations of identity possibilities available for citation and re-configuration of selfhood.

Our third digital mechanism implicated in the affordances of digital media for the revised taxonomy of gender and sexuality involves the very contemporary role of social networking as a central site for the performance of identity. The relationship is a complex one (Cover 2012b), although we can make some sense of it by thinking through the interface between interactivity as a mode of engagement and performativity as that which constitutes our identities, subjectivities and senses of selfhood. Indeed, social networking is a site through which identities are both articulated purposefully and wilfully through our contribution of profile information, self-selected image uploads and participation in conversations. It is, however, also a site by which our identities are put in question, engaged with and tested for their coherence and intelligibility, particularly through persistent conversation, 'likes' (or failures to like) and replies, responses and taggings from friends, family and others. All of these complexify and alter how our identities are represented and articulated.

At the same time, and as with all identity performativity, this also leaves us open to seeing the inherent flaw – that repetition of the signifiers we cite and the extension of our identities over time are doomed to failure, showing up on critical examination precisely how constructed and unstable identity can be. Social networking is a master site for this breakdown of identity coherence over time, because our timelines and feeds not only present a story of ourselves but also present us in all our inconsistencies, demanding an impossible extent of labour to truly and effectively 'shore up' our identities as unified, unchanging, coherent and recognisable. This is one space in which the coherence of heterosexual and homosexual, masculine and feminine identity categories becomes available for critique in a digital media setting. What is fostered in this setting is not only an intensive self-reflective relationship with identity through the demands of both profile development and engagement with those who are engaging with that profile but also an opportunity for the 'flaws' in identity performativity to emerge. So, when a lesbian identity becomes 'broken' in an online setting because the coherence of that identity is not maintained across a Facebook timeline, for example (perhaps by evidence of desiring the 'wrong way', or failing to conform to an expected stereotype), then it is highlighted in a way which is also semi-public. What this has done, then, is draw attention to the public and private *need* for a better way of describing gender and sexual identity to prevent such slippages from emerging in the face of others on our Facebook newsfeeds. And the responsive strategies, of course, have included fostering the search for better categories (for example heteroflexible, demigirl, etc.) that help shore up identity coherence.

Fourthly and finally, the one most significant aspect of digital media that might have actively enabled the challenge to current and received identity norms is the fact that digital media has brought together voices of those who may not necessarily have found an easy 'fit' with dominant gender (masculine/feminine) and sexuality (hetero/homo) normativities. The Internet plays a significant and continuing role in connecting disaffected persons to each other in ways that give access to and produce new experiential knowledges (Byron 2015, p. 324). According to critic Lenore Bell, the fact that these new identity labels emerged first on Tumblr may be due to the fact that its unique format is more removed from the everyday real life social networks than sites such as Facebook. Tumblr's network of friends is typically less likely to be made up of those known in geographic, physical senses, and more through bringing together those who are "connected by interests, and are not bound by personal interactions in real life . . . tailored to the individual reader's interests" (Bell 2013, p. 33). However, I would argue (again) that we need to be very careful not to assume too great a disjuncture between online settings of networked communities and 'real' communities produced through concepts of geographic locality: the distinction is complex and the interconnections between the two are multiple.

Certainly, however, digital media has been responsible for forging communities of disaffected persons in ways which have allowed the production of new knowledges, languages and sensibilities, often thereby empowering those communities in the act of creatively discussing alternatives that make lives more liveable for those who find themselves unrepresented. At the same time, the networked environment also provides those individuals and communities with voices that can actively challenge the dominant, the expert-derived discourses and information that represent monolithic, narrow, binary-based identity regimes that exclude or fail to represent in a meaningful way and have often left possibly quite large numbers of people feeling that the available categories are too narrow, regimentary, constraining and unliveable. By making available spaces for disparate people who feel unrepresented by dominant discourses, digital networks afford the production of new identities and ways of experiencing selfhood and relationality.

A prominent example over the past decade of the role digital networked communities play involves the way in which the 'Furry' community developed. Furries are a subculture within science fiction and fantasy fandom, and practices involve dressing as non-human anime characters. While this is often theatrics and not necessarily about a bodily dysmorphia (Dobre 2012), the identification as a Furry – that is, as a person whose sense of selfhood is defined by the engagement in such play – is deeply felt, an attachment that is subjective and performative. Such play, of course, may involve more serious identification with animals themselves, as some choose to live lives in an everyday sense through the theatrics of being a wolf or a cat (Dobre 2012). The Furry community and the construction of identity did not simply emerge by itself, but came about through the gathering online of very dispersed voices of those interested in this particular activity, forging a language and a shared sense of community.

Bearing in mind that all communities, whether begun online or in geographical or affiliational settings, precede the identities they claim to gather and are thereby 'imagined' into existence (Anderson 1983, pp. 6–7), it is through the development and sharing of symbolic frameworks of identity (Cohen 1985, p. 76) that a shared language is constructed. In so doing, the discourse for a new identity is articulated. The Furry community example is a useful one because it demonstrates how digital networking and the formation of 'virtual' communities play a significant role in the impetus of a new identity label and the codes of practices that make that label intelligible, available for citation, and iterable. The conditions that make a Furry community and label possible are the same conditions that permit the new taxonomy of gender and sexuality terms to be constituted.

Sexual citizenship

While digital media, then, is a site which makes available the space for the critique of gender and sexual identity norms and for both the dissemination and co-creation of alternative discourses, it does not in itself cause these but rather enables a cultural response to existing needs, gaps, exclusions, unliveabilities and other shortcomings in the dominant, liberal frameworks of binary-based gender and sexual identity models. I would therefore like to turn attention across the remainder of this chapter to the five key factors which help us understand those shortcomings and which have sponsored the development of the new taxonomy, beginning with the rise of sexual citizenship as a recent framing for contemporary sexuality. Sexual citizenship is a cultural and discursive re-conceptualisation of sexuality in ways which appear to encourage the agency of self-definition in the terms of personal and collective identities built on individualised perspectives of sexual attributes in order to claim recognition, rights and respect (Weeks 1998, p. 36). Sexual citizenship is a concept usually used to make sense of the intersection between sexuality, gender and sexual experiences and the political, social and cultural milieu in which sexuality is practiced. It permits sexuality and identity to be understood in terms of a struggle for rights and protections (Evans 1993), and for the idea of sexuality therefore to operate at the interface between the private (the domestic setting) and the public (the rights and relationality setting).

By providing a way to perceive the contemporary cultural representations and lived experiences of sexuality (Johnson 2017), a citizenship framework re-figures how sexuality is done, bringing into concepts of sexuality the private aspects of lived experienced as well as simultaneously privatising and domesticating sexual issues and making them in some ways external to the institutional settings of public life. It is thus responsible for the establishment of same-sex marriage rights and the movement seeking marriage equality (Dreher 2017), and for what has sometimes been felt to be a normativisation of non-heterosexualities and non-traditional genders, such that both the exclusions from national, public or institutional life for sexual minorities and, simultaneously, the marginalisation of anti-establishment Gay Liberation and queer politics of the past occurs in favour of the inclusion of sexuality into ordinary, everyday belonging. In this context, then, the sexual minorities defined through the ordinary, dominant terminology of LGBT identities are encouraged "to define themselves both in terms of personal and collective identities by their sexual attributes, and to claim recognition, rights and respect as a consequence" (Weeks 1998, p. 36). This does not mean that sexuality is no longer permitted to transgress but rather that transgression becomes instead a "constant invention and reinvention of new senses of the self" that challenge dominant institutions and traditions but are *only* subversive in the sense that they generate demands for belonging rather than an undoing of norms (Weeks 1998, p. 36). That subversion is, arguably, an output of productive engagement with questions of subjectivity, identity and gender/sexuality within a contemporary neoliberal imperative to produce the self through individualised reflexivity, selectivity and promotion to produce the "best possible" contemporary self – which in social terms is usually a conformative self.

If it has been the case to provide the dominant LGBT regime with a normativity, or what has sometimes been referred to as a homonormativity, producing new exclusions for those who are unable to conform to the contemporary, de-politicised sexuality labels (Duggan 2002), then what relationship does sexual citizenship play in the production of new genders and sexualities? Why is it not enough that a liberal tolerance setting for LGBT sexualities and genders does not provide sufficient belonging for liveable lives? One aspect of this is the fact that sexual citizenship is a neoliberal framing of sexuality and gender, and neoliberalism operates by the subsumption of *everything* into market relationships, while generating a market logic as the way in which to determine and understand *everything*. In other words, sexual citizenship undoes what it achieved for LGBT authenticity because it effectively seeks new opportunities in the gaps and interstices for marketisation.

Consumption and consumerism are increasingly playing a role in the general shift in the construction of identity and the performance of identity categories, in contrast to a more strict, broadly felt perception of "inner authenticity" or belonging centred on kinship ties and geographic community. Consumption is understood as the means by which subjectivity is grounded, felt and articulated in late contemporary capitalist cultures (Jameson 1985). Through surveillance, marketing and representation, contemporary culture plays a central role in processes of normativisation and measurement that differ from the disciplinary function of categorised norms such as those which produce the more simplistic hetero/homo and normal/abnormal binaries. Rather, a neoliberal framing that mutually 'services' both the market and governance technologies of biopolitics (Foucault 2008) calls upon subjects to *plot* their sense of normativity as points on a broader distributional curve, allowing some flexibility to move away from the culturally given norm (Foucault 2007, p. 63). In that sense, subjects are produced in this framework not through normal (heterosexual) and abnormal (homosexual, bisexual) distinctiveness, nor through superior (masculine; public) and inferior (feminine; domestic) dichotomies. As long as subjects do not stray too far from the norm on a measurable distributional curve, the broader range of new taxonomic terms and labels more effectively allows governance to capture the information on which it depends for its own logical existence, and the market to capture, target and produce a broader range of identity positions.

The practices of individual subjective production, circulation and consumption serve to encourage, foster and promote neoliberalism's particular regime of truth such that it subsumes *ways of thinking in all other fields aside from the economic*. This framework includes ways of thinking about the self, subjectivity and identity, which "involves generalising it throughout the social body and including the whole of the social system not usually conducted through or sanctioned by monetary exchanges" (Foucault 2008, p. 243). Every social and identity activity falls under the framework of an economic rationality, including the governance of the self (Foucault 2008, p. 286). Within this framework, the *homo oeconomicus* or "economic man" is produced. This is not, for Foucault, the classical economic man who is understood to be a partner in exchange. Rather, this is a neoliberal re-modelling of the subject as that which manages itself within the bounds of the biopolitical and the economic as an *investment* – one is an entrepreneur of selfhood and invests in one's own production of subjectivity (Foucault 2008, p. 226)

Important here, then, is the fact that for *homo oeconomicus* to produce oneself as not only a subject but also a gendered and sexual subject requires engaging with a *marketplace* of sexual and gender categories. In this context, a broader range of gender and sexuality labels can be said to have become available as a felt response to the contemporary neoliberal call for *choice*: a subject seeks to produce oneself through finding and choosing the most *productive* way of describing/articulating sexual selfhood, where older models based on hetero/homo categorical exclusivity are unproductive in that they require intensive conversational explanatory frameworks. In other words, a logic of consumption operates, not as if choosing an outfit but as choosing how subjectivity will be perceived and articulated, pivoting between self-authenticity as a response to the call for coherence and agency as a response to the call for a deeper level of authenticity. That is, my gender and my sexuality are to be seen to *come from me*, even if the only way in which they can come from me is by giving the impression of participating in choosing. Labels such as 'sapiosexual' or 'agender demisexual' are not only part of the range of choice but are also productive in that they allow a potentially more efficient stereotype of sexual identity to be enunciated in a few words rather than a longer explanation of complex sexual specificity – an *economisation* of sexual "explanatory" discourse. And, importantly, the subject then has consumed those labels in an economic exchange in which the labour of subjectivity is exchanged for the purchase of that which coheres sexual identity (and, of course, leaves the subject free to go on to be an even better consumer).

This is a very pessimistic perspective, of course, on the cultural factors that constitute the new taxonomy. What matters here, however, is that sexual citizenship provides some very powerful and useful ways in which to encourage a more liveable society for those who – for whatever reason – are unable to identify with dominant norms. Yet at the same time, sexual citizenship is both a product of and in service to prevailing biopolitical governance technologies and to neoliberal marketisation. By producing a greater range of labels that helps in identification and liveability, it produces a greater range of *products* to consume in a society in which *homo oeconomicus* is the dominant logic. The older relationships between anti-capitalism and anti-heteronormativity are shattered (Altman 1979, p. 64), and a proliferation of labels, identities and ways of relating mirrors the demands for economic growth. In this context, perhaps the link between labels as identifiers of goods on shelves and our identity labels is an apt one.

Cults of authenticity and personhood

Although some aspects of neoliberal sexual citizenship disrupt or destabilise the older, dominant LGBT norms, they do not quite produce a fluidity – partly for the reasons described above, in that they are not measurable in governance terms and not identifiable within the application of a transactional market logic to sexuality and gender. However, another reason for this is perhaps best talked about as being the appeal of 'authenticity'. What I sometimes refer to as a 'cult of authenticity' continues to govern the contemporary production of the performative self, a self who responds to the cultural demand for coherence, intelligibility and recognisability in order to participate socially and to belong. Authenticity is a very important aspect of this requirement for coherence, for without authenticity, the subject is open to the accusation of incoherence, and therefore of being perceived as schizophrenic, abject, or inhuman. It is, of course, the case that the language that constructs the categories of sex, gender, bodies and sexuality is by no means stable, but changes, reacts to the "making available" of alternative languages – such as emergent sexuality labels – and undergoes sometimes disruptive shifts in the logic on which that discourse is founded. In that context, there is no possible genuine authenticity of identity. Rather, we are all always already from the beginning doomed to perform our identities against the failure of coherence and intelligibility, since no true repetition of ourselves over time is possible.

An important argument here, however, is that the older, dominant labels of sexuality and gender are more likely to produce problems of authenticity and coherence. This is for a few reasons. In the sexual setting of hetero and homo, the identity categories are old enough that there is enough evidence at both personal and social levels for us to know that the connection between the category on the one hand and the expected behaviours, attractions and desires on the other hand is not very secure at all. Indeed, everyday humour, suspicions, experiences and even acceptances of slippage occur. It is in the radical failure of the self-containedness of the two categories of heterosexual and homosexual that the new taxonomy of sexualities emerges, for the rather simple reason that it is very difficult for many people to perform a coherent and unified heterosexuality or homosexuality once the diffuse potentiality of complex sexual desire, erotic attachment, or romantic engagement is taken into account. Indeed, as Butler has noted, repetition is core to the project of articulating a coherent identity (Butler 1990, pp. 31–32); a repetition of stylised acts gives intelligibility over time (pp. 140–141), offering a retroactive sense of an inner identity core (p. 136). Repetition is, in a poststructuralist framework, always marked by its own internal potentiality of failure: an *exact* reiteration is impossible, and this can include the reiteration of a sex act, a desire or, most pertinently here, an identification. While Butler's early work proposed a kind of forgetting or "unthinkability" (Butler 1990, p. 77) of the failure to repeat the performance of subjecthood properly over time, it might be argued that, today, there is a greater awareness of the 'work' of identity as a laborious process (p. 70) in which there is a far greater realisation of being doomed to fail under categories that are too broad, too complex or, as with hetero- and homo-sexualities, in which there are too many known instances of the failure to repeat (a sex act, a desire, an identification) properly.

In this context, then, the imperative for authenticity in light of the failure of the hetero/homo distinction to operate seamlessly for all subjects results in a cultural demand for more complex categories through which subjects can perform an identity that, illusively, appears or feels *more authentic*. New sexualities, then, can be understood as identifications with labels through which one can account for the anomalies of attractions that run counter to the stereotyped logic of the labels heterosexual or homosexual, even though they continue to use the identity language and coming out practices of older sexualities. A wider range of categories answers the call for sexual identity authenticity. It provides a greater range of labels with *nuance*. The term 'greysexual' is an excellent example. It overcomes the possibility of a subject being identified on one side or another of a well-policed border in a new dichotomy of 'sexual' versus 'nonsexual', where a *border crossing* would decimate authenticity. That is, the avowed asexual who has, in the right circumstances, a sexual experience, cannot authentically be asexual. The greysexual person, where the term incorporates the occasional possibility of sexual expression, experience, desire or attraction, can be open to it and experience it without the accusation – that might come equally from oneself as from another – that one was not *truly asexual* to begin with.

Heteroflexible and homoflexible are other such identity terms that provide authenticity to sexual subjectivity. Where a slippage in heterosexuality or homosexuality casts suspicion (again, perhaps just as likely to come for the self as another), the authenticity of one's heterosexual identity has been known to become suspect in the latter half of the twentieth century. Eric Anderson (2008) has referred to the 'one-time rule' in which a single same-sex sexual encounter, or slip-up or articulated albeit unfulfilled desire will charge a heterosexual man, in some circumstances, with having always been gay, or having now changed to become gay. In gay male culture of the late-twentieth century, an avowedly gay man who has a sexual encounter with a woman has been at risk of being referred to as a 'traitor'. In both cases, the inference is that they are not *authentically* straight or gay. The terms heteroflexible and homoflexible, however, allow those who might have an occasional 'dalliance' outside of the strictures of heterosexual or homosexual expectations to be able to use an identity label that represents their experience more authentically rather than being (mis)recognised as a non-authentic heterosexual or homosexual. In other words, the new taxonomy provides opportunities for representing the self as an authentic self.

So, our second 'causal factor' is the fact that there is a deep cultural desire for authenticity and the broad set of micro-minoritised identity labels are more efficient and effective in providing authenticity for the reasons I have just described. Why, however, does authenticity matter? While I would prefer to opt for a sociality in which temporal coherence was not a key requirement for intelligible subjectivity, it remains that there is a deep desire to feel secure in one's subjectivity. Authenticity is central to generating that affect. Butler (1997) pointed to the fact there must at play be a *desire for subjection*, in the sense of the way in which Althusser's interpellation is a giving over to the rule of an ideology or discourse. She asked if it might be the case that there is a simple "love of the shackles" that constrain us into narrow, fixed, essentialist identity categories of gender and sexuality, and determined that the desire for subjection is a matter of the desire for existence (p. 27). That is, the regimes of power actively require subjection *to categories of identity themselves* in order to continue as a recognisably coherent and authentic social being. If we consider authenticity as a form of identity fixity over time, a disavowal of being one's identity's other, and an engagement in the 'hard labour' of policing one's actions, experiences, desires. attractions and wishes in order stay within the bounds of the identity category, then it remains important to recognise that this is done for the very sake of existence. Those who can disavow authenticity, however, need a grounding (as a broad-based critical label like queer), an alternative discourse (such as poststructuralist queer theory) and the skills in articulating that critical perspective in order to maintain, in Butler's term, survival and existence. Our need for existence as a subject is thus central to the need for a broader taxonomic range of identity and gender labels through which subjects can better avoid 'inauthentic' lives.

Labelling the gaps and responding to the abyss

With the above points in mind, it is worth thinking about what kinds of unliveabilities might have been experienced by those who, in the older, dominant discourse of hetero/homo and masculine/feminine categorical authenticity, were unable to present themselves in alignment with the available categories. In *Queer Youth Suicide, Culture and Identity: Unliveable Lives?* (2012a), I wrote about some of the ways in which we might understand queer youth suicide through alternative cultural studies approaches, primarily to respond to the question that if homophobia was a cause of sexuality-related suicide, why does the rate remain relatively the same over time when there has been a substantial implementation of social support and a very significant shift towards a liberal–tolerant society. A few of the other ways of thinking about the causes of suicidality included looking at relative disparities in happiness among those identifying as LGBT, where 'relative misery' among a community is a known suicide cause in some sociological scholarship; the way shame might be understood to persist despite liberal tolerance, where shame is a perceive suicide causal factor in some older scholarship; and the over-regimentation of sexual identities, where regimentation and regulation appear in Emile Durkheim's (1952) account of suicide causes and whereby some people feel like life is unliveable because they fall through the gaps and are unable to present themselves authentically within the given, narrow, regimented categories of heterosexual and homosexual.

The notable matter here is the question of 'gaps' – of what it means not to be represented and what the inability to be recognised as a subject does for liveability. Understanding the debilitating effects of the gaps between how one might 'feel' one's identity to be and the regimentary expectations of what is expected is significant for making sense of why there has been such substantial interest in a new taxonomy of identity labels that better represent those gaps and provide identity intelligibility for those who fall into the gaps. One question that is sometimes raised in relation to this point is this: if identity is performative, and it is given in discourse through a process of subjection, then how is it possible a person can feel that they are outside those discourses unless identity was always from the beginning determined biologically, genetically, at the level of the body? Such an argument would, of course, be to try and find an answer to essentialist/constructionist debates by coming to one side or the other. Although identity is constituted in discourse (in the available languages and cultural norms and practices), a wholly culturally determinist perspective on identity formation was certainly never the intention of Butler (1993), who pointed out that a radical constructionist perspective was just as dangerous as those discourses which argued for a wholesale biological or genetic essentialism to identity, particularly but not exclusively in relation to gender and sexuality. Both miss the point and the value of deconstruction (p. 8). Rather, the alternative is to understand that bodies, desire, genders and *felt* ways of being operate across different languages and registers each for us, even though we are required to disavow that complexity in favour of authenticity. Those who cannot disavow, then, are at risk – not necessarily of being accused of being incoherent or unintelligible, but of perceiving life to be unliveable if the affectively felt sense of self and the regimentary categories one is required to perform are at a mis-match.

For those who, for whatever reason, are unable to forge a deep sense of 'fit' with the available categories of gender and sexuality or are unable to perform coherently within those dominant categories over a protracted period of time, there is a consequential risk that imperils the ability to be recognised by others. As Butler (2005) notes,

> to question the norms of recognition that govern what I might be, to ask what they leave out, what they might be compelled to accommodate, is, in relation to the present regime, to risk unrecognisability as a subject or at least to become an occasion for posing the questions of who one is (or can be) and whether or not one is recognizable.
>
> *(p. 23)*

What this means, and what has concerned me from a health, mental health and wellbeing perspective, is that there is potentially a very significant difference between the one who finds the failure of recognition to be an occasion for questions about identity, and the one who is stranded in unrecognisability and incoherence. It is a matter of the uneven distribution of skills in critique, which is not to say that this uneven distribution aligns with other kinds of inequitable resource distribution, whether education, financial, racial or in terms of geography, mobility or age. Rather, what it means is that while some thrive in the face of a moment in non-recognition that, in interpellative terms, hails or calls upon us to rethink (to recognise) subjecthood by seeking out a new, alternative discourse or framing that provides intelligibility, others are positioned into an unliveability, because contemporary liberal–humanist culture persists in the underlying, base requirement for coherent, intelligible and recognisable identities. In other words, not being in a position to find an alternative grounding in order to perform and perceive oneself as a coherent and recognisable subject by questioning, critiquing or resisting the violence of social regulation or over-regulation is to risk *access to subjectivity*, social participation and belonging, to risk exclusion from intelligibility and selfhood. Naturally, where unintelligibility centres on questions of deeply held norms related to gender identity and the coherence of sexual orientation patterns played out over time, these risks tend to become exacerbated in ways that tend to be less prominent for other coordinates or categories of identity. And where unintelligibility and inability to be recognised *as a subject* (or to recognise oneself as a subject) in whatever terms are available become unliveable, suicide is one of the logics by which many continue to be respond to the unbearable, intolerable affect of unliveability (Shneidman 1985, p. 36; Kral 1994).

So what, then, might make possible a gap between how one 'feels' as a gendered or sexual subject and the available discourses? I would like to say a few words about how this might be understood, since it is not simply a matter of assuming the available discourse (whether the dominant binary discourses or the new taxonomy) will *exhaustively* constitute the subjects it purports to name. Rather, we need to understand the fact that there is a body at play – not a body that is genetically predisposed to desire one way or another or that is determinedly male or female, since such ideas are only legible and readable in *the terms of the available discourse*. Rather, the body of the subject is a body that can have aspects of performance, biology, attachment, parts, desires and ways of being that cannot be translated into the logic of the dominant discourse. For example, the body that feels itself androgynous or intersexed and cannot be shoe-horned into a category of masculinity or femininity. Or the body that affectively feels it desires in a way that does not conform to heterosexual, homosexual or bisexual regimentations.

We can think of this 'feltness' as a kind of bodily 'residue' of all that which is unassimilable to discourse in the process of an embodied subject materialising into a particular gender or sexual subjectivity. Such a concept of residue operates in a conceptually similar way to the Lacanian notion of *jouissance* – what Elizabeth Grosz (1989), following Irigaray, sees as a *remainder* "left unrepresented in a phallic libidinal economy" (p. 115). This is not necessary something we can assimilate to a mind/body dualism in which the mind has one identity and the body the other; rather, this is the unrepresentable in the context of the body that is materialised as a *product of culture* (Grosz 1994, p. 55). In our case, that is a product of gender and sexual discourses and the cultural demands for coherent, intelligible and recognisable genders and sexualities, whether in accord with dominant categories or alternative ones. The body as an animate organisation of flesh, muscle and tissue is, of course, always biologically "incomplete" to begin with (Grosz 1995, p. 104). Within that process of materialisation and subjection to discourse we can find the residue of that which is not made intelligible material. What I am thus arguing here is that there can be bodily aspects that feel like they rub against gender the wrong way or don't seem to work in a discursive gender framework, and there can be libidinal or erotic sensibilities or desires that remain unassimilable by the discourses that demand coherent orientations. In other words, at the site of the materialisation of the body into a coherent, culturally representable gendered and sexualised body, there are non-materialised residues that cannot be reconfigured or reconstituted *in accord* with the discourses of gender and sexuality. Obviously, this may change if different, new, alternative, emergent discourses are made available or, indeed, stumbled on, providing ways of recognising one's gender or sexual subjectivity and assimilating such a residue into a seemingly more coherent, intelligible and socially recognisable self. No subjectivity, of course, is totalised fully – what matters is that a coherent performativity depends upon the illusion of authenticity and totality – being totally masculine or totally feminine, for example, according to the older, dominant discourse in its most demanding and regimentary setting.

So, what use is this bodily 'residue' that upsets the possibility of performing *as if* a totalised subject within the contemporary cultural demands for subjects answerable as subjects? Is it external to language in a way which might provide a radical desta-bilisation of language itself? Possibly not. Butler is uncertain about the possibility of an exterior to language. She suggests that to "posit by way of language a materiality outside of language is still to posit that materiality, and the materiality so posited will retain that positing as its constitutive condition" (Butler 1993, p. 30). She goes on to point out that language is not opposed to materiality, as if in some dichotomy between the body and culture; at the same time, embodied materiality itself cannot simply be collapsed into languages of identity (p. 68). Nevertheless, for Butler, there is indeed a kind of 'outside' to what is constructed by discourse:

> this is not an absolute 'outside', [but] an ontological there-ness that exceeds or counters the boundaries of discourse; as a constitutive 'outside', it is that which can only be thought – when it can – in relation to that discourse, at and as its most tenuous borders.
>
> *(p. 68)*

Thus, any outside or exterior is always constituted in terms of the interior – it can only ever be known and imagined through the discourses available to us in the interior. This makes it difficult to bear witness to the 'residue' that is unassimilable to discourse and that, for some, may make an authentic performance of gender or sexual subjectivity untenable.

However, there are ways in which we can conceptually frame the idea of a 'space' in which a *particular* language or discourse has no entry, and thereby is unable to assimilate that which does not 'fit' in a cultural regime of gender and sexuality within the old dominant discourse prior to the new taxonomy. Jacques Derrida's theorisation of the *khora* (or 'chora') is helpful in this regard. For Derrida (1989), the chora as a receptacle or container can be thought; it is itself a concept that can be signified in language and discourse, but what it *contains* cannot. The chora signifies a place that "belongs neither to the sensible nor to the intelligible, neither to becoming, nor to non-being (the *khora* is never described as a void)" (p. 36) that can only ever be described a "bastard reasoning" (pp. 34–35). What the chora contains is that which cannot be reasoned or understood in the *available* discourse – it is the unsignifiable and the unknowable, and that can include both *felt* but *unintelligible* to an individual subject on the basis of the discourses available to that subject, implying it may well be intelligible in terms of other discourses that are presently *unavailable* to that particular subject. Thus, the chora is situated beyond the margins of an available discourse. Or, to be more clear, that which at a particular time for a particular person, society, culture or knowledge regime is unrepresentable, or for which identity classifications, names and signifiers do not (yet) exist.

To give an example, we could think about this in the case of, say, a subject whose gender identity might be read through the new taxonomy as 'nobi-sexual' (defined as having fluctuating or fluid gender feelings that are limited to genders either neutral and/or neither masculine or feminine – that is, movement around gender identification that does not at any stage fall into either masculine or feminine). That is fine for those us with access to a discourse that makes such gender complexity, malleability and movement intelligible, and either the new taxonomy or poststructuralist critiques of the power/knowledge framework of gender or discourses of androgyny can provide this stability, coherence, authenticity and grounding. However, what about for the subject who feels their gender is in some way moving about in this particular space, a little fluid, a little changeable but not quite either masculine or feminine? What if that subject has available to them *only* the dominant discourse that articulates gender as compulsorily masculine/feminine? Then that felt experience of being something other than the genders prescribed by the dominant, available discourse is relegated to the chora – felt, but unsayable; there is no language to make this gender understood.

Alternatively, in the context of sexuality and eros, a subject might have a felt experience of polymorphous diffusion of eros across the body that is unrelated to gender, to the genitals and to engaging with other bodies *as gendered bodies*. Indeed, such polymorphous perversity is, in much psychoanalytic discourse, perceived to be the universal human experience albeit repressed (Freud 1979, p. 178) and refocused in adulthood onto the genitals to relegate sexual expression to the domestic sphere and to ensure the body operates most effectively as an instrument of labour (Marcuse 1969). Such polymorphous perversity is very much sexual and erotic and may be felt at a point that denies repression; yet again it may be unassimilable to the dominant discourses of sexuality that prescribe a compulsory identification as coherent heterosexual, homosexual or bisexual and instead relegated to the chora. It is *experienced*, but as with much self-experience it is not accessed in a way that can be adequately described in the available languages (Belsey 1994, p. 10). Rather, it remains inaccessible to ourselves, although it may perhaps be readable and interpretable in some cases by those with access to alternative discourses. Indeed, for Derrida (1989), what occurs in the chora is an 'experience' that is "above all *not* an experience, if one understands by this word a certain presence, whether it is sensible or intelligible or even a relation to the presence of the present in general" (pp. 38–39). Thus, what might be experienced in that space in a particular subject is a particular felt experience of gender or of sexuality that is *beyond* thinkability within certain discourses available, even if this might have intelligibility in discourses not yet available to that subject.

If such experiences are to be located in the chora, which is not in itself a site of repression but a container for that which cannot be articulated in a discourse, then does it actually matter? For the subjects as I am describing them: yes. It matters because the disjuncture between cultural demand for coherent gender and sexuality, and the bodily residue of an alternative but deeply felt sense of gender or sexual selfhood (that may not necessarily yet be quite the same as subjectivity), can establish an inability *to be* in society, to articulate oneself in a recognisable way, even if one does not quite know why.

One way we can think of the problem as that which causes stresses, anxieties, suicidalities, unliveabilities and so on – at least in some subjects who may not have had the benefit of access to a broader range of gender/sexuality discourses – is through the geographic notion of a chasm. The bodily residue of the felt experience and the available or dominant discourses can be thought of as 'located' across a *chasm of non-translatability* between the two: a chasm of the impossibility of assimilation or recognition, preventing the subject from achieving the culturally demanded requirements of coherence, intelligibility and authenticity. The fact that this is located in the chora is what ensures there is no possibility of *translation* between the choral desire and the codes of gender or sexuality as they are known. What is in the chora 'speaks' a language, but one which cannot be understood; it is part of the languages of the "unsayable" (Budick and Iser 1989, p. XI). What it requires, then, is translation. Unfortunately in a poststructuralist perspective, translation itself is fundamentally impossible, as the act of translation demands a substitution or transformation of signifiers that are accessible (Derrida 1978, p. 210). Discourse cannot translate that which is in the chora, as it remains 'untouchable' to the signification in translation (Derrida 1985, p. 114). What we thus have in the chora is a set of felt experiences which are *monolingual*. While dominant discourses, as we know from Butler (1990), attempt to impose their categories and thereby re-configure the subject as a particular type of subject, their attempts to translate and capture these affectively felt bodily residues are simultaneously colonial in style and practice. Colonising the experience of otherness occurs in the act of language to reduce language to a singularity, or towards what Derrida (1996) refers to as the "hegemony of the homogeneous" (pp. 39–40). Since the logic of that which is within the chora is not intelligible to the colonising discourse, the experiences, desires and affects it contains remain unassimilable.

What then for the subject who has no available alternative discourse with which to make intelligible those deeply felt and sensed residues located in the chora into an expressible, speakable, performative subjectivity? The untranslatability of that which is contained in the chora (bodily desire, experience of desire; desires which cannot be understood in dominant terms) is what I refer to as the *chasm*. While it is plausible that a subjectivity can be performed in disavowal of the dominant (binary) codes of gender and sexuality, what is required is an alternative set of discursive codes which might bridge a translation across this chasm between the subject who is subjected to what is in the chora and the contemporary dominant hetero/homo discourse. This is necessary, because without the attempt to fulfil the social injunction *to be*, no subject is socially intelligible and must thereby be relegated to the margins. A discursive platform is necessary: a defence. In the case of a chora-located experience of gender and sexuality, we might find that Freudian polymorphous perversity is one *suitable* code that can bridge the chasm and translate the experience into that which is performable *as subject*, even if in opposition to the fixed, linear and categorical genital-focused sexuality and gender definitions of the dominant. A radical, albeit marginal, queer politics of fluidity might be another that provides a suitable grounding for that felt experience or sense of otherness, allowing a performance that meets the requirements of coherence, intelligibility and recognisability – even if the field of recognition is a marginal one located in alternative cultures. *This is to assume that such discourses can and will be available to a subject.*

Suicide, mental health concerns, breakdown, dislodged social participation and other ways of being positioned as 'unhealthy' are what otherwise occur without a sensible, suitable discourse through which to make these residues of the contained otherness intelligible. I have previously discussed (Cover 2012a) some of the ways in which identity regimentation – and its failure – can be understood to lead to suicidality in certain cases and under certain conditions, including those described above. To exaggerate the chasm metaphor into the trope of the abyss, we can note John Caputo's association of the abyss with suicide and the breakdown of coherent selfhood. For Caputo (1993), suicide occurs because the abyss is both an unknowability and a knowability in which the subject is "cut off from the comforts of a deep and reassuring ground" (p. 329), which in our case means to be cut off from an available discourse that presents an explanatory framework for a nuanced gender or sexuality to the world and, most particularly, to oneself.

With the context of this scenario in mind, I am arguing that the new taxonomy is – in part – an emergent response to the abject failure of the dominant, binary-based discourses of masculinity and femininity, to the heterosexual matrix and to both homophobic and liberal–tolerant discourses to provide a grounding for everyone, building ways to avoid the chasm and to ensure that which is relegated to the chora as the unintelligible sensibility of gender or sexuality is speakable and representable. It is a response that attempts to account for *diversity*, and particularly then for and on behalf of those who fall between the cracks, those whose felt sense of subjectivity leaves them unable to be a subject answerable as a subject, those who see themselves looking into the chasm or into the abyss of suicidality, because the inability to articulate one's gender or one's sexuality with coherence leaves life unliveable. Providing labels that address the possibility of a felt sense that does not conform to or is unassimilable by the dominant, masculine/feminine and hetero/homo frameworks presents the possibility of avoiding the abyss, of allowing that which is contained and untranslatable to speak in a way which has coherence and intelligibility in performativity and thus cross that chasm. And, finally, while other discourses might have done a similar job – including Freudian polymorphous perversity, the androgyny in popular culture of the 1970s, radical discourses of Gay Liberation, avant-garde anti-establishmentarian critiques, poststructuralist queer theory of the 1990s – the new taxonomy does a better and more efficient job, precisely because unlike the others it does not question coherence, intelligibility and identity themselves which risk leaving many feeling groundless. Rather, it, leaves the cultural imperative of authentic subjecthood intact while presenting a greater schema or range of categories, classifications and labels of genders and sexualities through which to be authentic and contained.

Disavowing fluidity: the underlying cultural demand of subjectivity

Our fourth explanatory framework for the emergence of the new taxonomy of classificatory terms relates somewhat more to the politics of some of the older debates in the 1990s between a more conservative, ethnic rights styled approach to LGBT rights that demanded a strategic use of coherent and consistent 'born that way' identities, and a queer politics that advocated an anti-establishment approach and an embrace of 'fluidity'. I described fluidity in Chapter 2 not in the everyday way that sometimes assumes genders and sexualities might be boundless, ever-changing, responsive to circumstance, like fluid moved into different vessels. For example, participants in Lisa Diamond's (2008) study of fluidity among women included participants who adopted the self-descriptor fluid because it was a better term than bisexuality for those who felt their attractions had nothing to do with desiring both genders *as genders* (p. 187). This is valuable; however, as a descriptor it recalls an individualism and an agency that is unhelpful in addressing cultural regimentations of categories.

Rather, fluidity in the poststructuralist sense I am using it in refers to the denaturalisation of the rigid categories as given in discourse, providing gender and sexuality with *contingency* and *historical temporality*. To invoke fluidity means to understand gender and sexuality as given in ways which are regimentary and constraining in discourse, and to acknowledge that the performances of identities may feel essential and natural but are effectively only illusions prescribed upon us so that we can meet the demands of intelligibility, authenticity and coherence in order to be subjects answerable as subjects. Fluidity also means to acknowledge relationality – the construction if identities according to categories and in ways which put subjectivity first are exclusionary. Relational approaches acknowledge that the I/You dichotomy (Game and Metcalfe 2011, p. 353) need not be oppositional, but that every identity forged is done so in the context of recognition and incorporation of the other rather than radically differentiating oneself from the other. A relational approach opens the possibility of a genuine mutuality that is more ethical in terms of engaging in a non-violent sociality. So, while fluidity has a complex set of meanings that take us down to the very kernel of subjectivity as culturally produced and regimented, much of the public assumption and negative critique of gender and sexual fluidity tends to focus on it in the more simplistic as boundless movement and change in an orgiastic frenzy of persistent instability.

The new micro-minority categorisations of gender and sexuality tend, in both their structure and much of their definitional content, not only to actively eschew the extant, older binary definitions but also to *reinforce* the force of categorisation and the public requirement for clear, coherent, intelligible and recognisable gender and sexual identities fixed over time. The demand for a more nuanced framework and taxonomy of labels is, arguably, in order to prevent any slippages that might undo the schemata of sexual labelling. That is, what they speak is that the older categorisations are not only unrepresentative, but precisely *because they are problematic* they are at risk of permitting slippages that do little for the underlying cultural requirements for *coherent* subjectivities – coherent within a category or bound. This reasoning, and the feelings underlying it, can most clearly be understood in thinking about the two identity categories of heteroflexible and homoflexible, which, themselves, have become two significant micro-minorities claiming rights for inclusion, often within an LGBT spectrum of sexual subjectivities. OkCupid describes the identity category homoflexible as "predominantly homosexual but open to an occasional heterosexual encounter". A crowdsourced comment from OkCupid user Katrina from Canada describes it in more personal terms: "Homoflexible means that while I am attracted to women generally, I am entirely capable of having sexy fun time with men" (www.okcupid.com/deep-end/identity/homoflexible). A heteroflexible orientation is unsurprisingly described in similar, but oppositional, terms: "Heteroflexibility is a form of a sexual orientation or situational sexual behaviour characterised by minimal homosexual activity in an otherwise primarily heterosexual sexual orientation that is considered to distinguish it from bisexuality" (www.okcupid.com/identity/heteroflexible). Notable in many such online descriptions, self-articulations and definitions of heteroflexibility and homoflexibility are the multiple affective terms such as *capable* (of experiencing same-sex sexual and erotic pleasure), *fantasies* (that may not necessarily be acted upon) and *infatuation* (that may not necessarily be of a "sexual" but "emotional" character). The terms homo- and heteroflexible distinguish a subject from bisexual, an orientation normatively described by OkCupid as "sexually attracted to both men and women" (www.okcupid.com/identity/homoflexible).

These labels, then, actively incorporate aspects of capability, nonsexual attachment and same gender or opposite gender fantasy *within* a category of sexual orientation, thereby overcoming the kinds of exclusions that have been produced by Anderson's (2008) 'one-time rule' (a cultural perception that a heterosexual man who has a sexual experience or fantasy about another man is thereby gay, even if that fact remained undisclosed to himself) and by same-sex masculine intimacy (in which masculine subjects can engage in same-sex kissing, hugging, or holding on condition these acts are stripped of all sexual connotation in public discourse). Heteroflexible and homoflexible sexual identity classifications address both of these ideas about masculine sexuality: they remove the 'one-time rule' from seeing a sexual encounter with the 'wrong' gender as *proving* a particular orientation or eradicating the previously claimed heterosexual identity on the one hand and, on the other, they restore sexuality and eroticism to same-sex relations.

An argument for the emergence of new practices of categorising sexualities such as the two 'flexible' labels is that they make existing dominant identity labels, such as heterosexual and homosexual, feel more secure. Rather than incorporating slippage or fluidity across categories, these new sexual identity labels actively reduce slippage by *assigning slippage itself* to particular subjects and to particular classifications, thereby reducing the possibility that either a heterosexual person or a homosexual person can 'slip', that is, that anyone is capable of finding themselves performing sexual or gendered selves, acts, attractions and desires different from those they thought they were classified within. In the twentieth-century regime of sexual identity distinctiveness, the hetero/homo binary operates as a "nodal point" which, as with many other binaries, actively prevents the *conceptual slippage* of the signified under the signifier (Mouffe 1995, p. 34), thus excluding alternatives to the hetero/homo regime as impossible articulations in cultural discourses. That is, in prior sexual regimes, homosexuality and heterosexuality were presumed to be mutually exclusive identities that were "totalised" against slippage. While Diana Fuss (1995) suggested that there is much evidence of the queer potential for multiple sexual identifications within the same subject which can compete with each other, "producing further conflicts to be managed" (p. 49), such conflict and nuance is responded to through the pretence that disavows complexity in favour of a sense of fixity, fixed orientation, and the 'totalisation' of that category across the entirety of a subject's being, stabilised across the entirety of that subject's life. As Foucault (1990) put it, there was a perception from the late nineteenth century that the "total composition" of a homosexual subject, for example, was marked by his homosexuality, "consubstantial with him, less as a habitual sin than as a single nature" (p. 43). That is, a subject – who is answerable in contemporary culture *as a subject*, is to be thought of not as a person who repeats, perhaps compulsively or unwittingly, a certain act, desire, attraction or feeling. Rather, he or she is framed as a personage, a full nature that does not permit change or movement, or to be also outside the categorical bound of a singular, unitary label.

The two key points here are that a regime of sexual categorisation has existed throughout the twentieth and twenty-first centuries as a way of managing conflict in subjectivity and regimenting the subject into a category, classification, name or signifier. Subjectivity *must* be performed with coherence, unity, intelligibility and recognisability across time. Multiplicity, confusion, curiosity and other more multifarious disruptions (or *fluidities*) are permissible only if they can be captured and re-subjectified. In that context, the proliferation of gender and sexual labels occurs as a *response* to the failure of the older, more narrow categories of heterosexual, homosexual and bisexual to account for and properly encapsulate sexual behaviour, gendered bodies, felt senses of selfhood and attraction and desire in totality.

Arguably, then, a broader set of categories or a grid of sexual identities operates to ensure that any slippage from heterosexual or homosexual is contained not as a "moment of weakness" or curiosity but as way of disavowing evidence of the unworkability of categories and labels of sexual identity. A more nuanced set of labels that will capture and subsume slippages is proffered, allowing flexibility without working outside the cultural demand for regimented, fixed and intelligible sexual subjectivities itself. The very force of the hetero/homo binary is overthrown as a nodal point in favour of ensuring sexual identity itself can remain essentialised against the "threat" of diversity and fluidity. When Butler (1990) called for a "radical proliferation of gender *to displace* the very gender norms that enable the repetition itself", she made clear that this was not merely a *propagation of categories* of gender that produce new identity norms in greater number, but a framework for moving beyond regimentary gendered ontologies since they "always operate within established political contexts as normative injunctions, determining what qualifies as intelligible sex, invoking and consolidating the reproductive constraints on sexuality" (p. 148). As Butler (1997) has put it, regulation impacts significantly on the liveability of the subject: "subjection is the paradoxical effect of a regime of power in which the very 'conditions of existence', the possibility of continuing as a recognisable social being, requires the formation and maintenance of the subject in subordination" (p. 27). Through processes of subjection and regulation, subjects are produced and required to perform, behave, and desire by maintaining and exploiting the cultural demand for "continuity, visibility, and place" (p. 29). That is, in the process of developing a sexual identity, young sexual subjects are culturally required to respond and "fit" within regulatory norms in order to fulfil the condition of existence through performing as a "recognizable social being" (Butler 1997, p. 27).

It is important not to prescribe these alternatives from within contemporary frameworks of sexuality and gender; in that respect, they may remain at least partly unknowable. As with the older regimentations of identity, the new taxonomy is marked by the fact that the subject answerable as subject remains *definitionally* built into each of the gender or sexual category labels, thereby articulating a classificatory system that is built not on relationality but individualism and exclusion. As Ken Plummer (1995) has remarked, there is a need to look for new stories that "take us beyond the limiting categories of the past" (p. 160). New stories that open the field of possibilities for inclusive sexualities must rely on a post-categorisational framing of sexuality through a concept of "fluidity", which is to hark back to one strand of Gay Liberation's proto-queer imperative for a liberation built on a "new diversity, an acceptance of the vast possibilities of human experience" (Altman 1971, p. 115). In the context of youth sexualities, Ritch Savin-Williams (2001) has produced a call for a framework for overcoming exclusions and producing new normativities by eschewing "sexual labels altogether and rely[ing] on descriptions of behaviours, desires or attractions" (p. 11). These arguments for fluidity are in stark contrast, then, from the activities of the taxonomy which operate to classify, regiment and curtail change, movement, slippage, criticism, anti-foundationalism and the desubjectification of the subject.

Fluidity is thus problematic for those who do not have the conceptual framework for thinking about the disruption of subjectivity itself. So, we might say that fluidity is actively disavowed because of the unconscious but culturally important need to shore up the subject. This disavowal of fluidity that underpins the new taxonomy is not necessarily expressed in those terms; indeed, as subjectivity is so deeply entrenched and de-naturalised, it is not necessarily evoked in its own defence. Rather, fluidity is sometimes critiqued because it is seen to contradict social and scientific implications built on notions of essentialism and genetics (Diamond 2008, p. 236) and sometimes argued against because it disrupts the ethnic 'civil rights' model that has been responsible for the hard-won gains towards tolerance and legal protections of coherently categorised LGBT subjects (Epstein 1990). Concepts of fluidity – whether those of the more pedestrian free-flowing identity conceptualisation or those of the poststructuralist critique of subjectivity – are also very often related to a concept of instability. Instability, as Mari Ruti (2017) has recently noted, is being increasingly understood by contemporary queer theory as a cause of suffering (p. 41). Ruti relates instability to some broader global conditions such as compulsory mobility, forced migration and other kinds of disruptions that make life unliveable. Indeed, this is poignant in that if a struggle for new gender and sexuality labels is a struggle to provide grounding, letting grounding shake, moving those grounds, is directly contra to the purposes at hand. Or we could think of instability as the spilling over that, in Mary Douglas (1966) terms, is required to remain separated in order to fulfil the affective desire for purity. The upsetting of the strictures of categories that an everyday account of fluidity produces, like the upsetting of subjectivity that a queer theoretical assertion of fluidity generates, is deeply upsetting at a constitutional level to subjects themselves. The taxonomy does an excellent job of re-stabilising and providing a more easily liveable order.

The role of populism and anti-expertise

All of the fluidity-advocating approaches outlined above are, obviously, exceedingly disruptive from the perspective of subjectivity. If the aim of those seeking better, more inclusive and more ethical ways to do gender and sexuality is just that – to find better ways of doing gender and sexuality – that is not the same as calling for new ways to do subjectivity, identity and selfhood *per se*. So while, as with many queer theorists, I might strongly desire that destabilisation and, indeed, argue that the radical critique of subjectivity itself would actually produce *even better* ways of doing gender and sexuality, the fact remains that a poststructuralist, critical and queer theoretical perspective is not necessarily shared by everyone, not necessarily accessible to everyone and not necessarily able to divorce itself from a particular kind of elitism which marks much scholarship and academic theory. In that context, we need to think not so much about there being different, competing ways in which to upset the dominant discourses of gender and sexuality – or, worse, to make value judgements about which one is the 'right' one. Rather, what is needed is understanding some of the reasons why the fluidity-advocating approaches are excluded (or shored-up against) by the new taxonomy.

In addition to the reasons for its cultural development that I have given above, a perspective on this would involve locating the entirety of the taxonomy-generating enterprise within a broad cultural populism that has emerged over the past decade across a range of spheres. Populism, then, is the fifth and last 'cause' that I would like to discuss here. Populism in recent years is very much associated with the rise of Donald Trump in the United States, supported by a vocal minority called the alt-right who have been very much focused on the criticism of 'the establishment' which is – somewhat ironically – seen to be at fault for being too dominated by a liberal elite, that is, upper-middle-class subjects who are in positions comfortable enough to be able to articulate social justice claims. A populist coalition has formed on a global scale which denounces liberal politics of migrant inclusion, LGBT rights, gender equality and anti-racism; this is a coalition built to include those who feel disenfranchised economically, those who see a political divide between urban culture and rural and suburban life and those in power positions who feel that their status is at risk of slipping, such as hegemonic articulations of masculinity. Some of the disenchantment is, of course, well-justified. The new populism is actually not at all new. The current mode seen in many anglophone countries is merely a new generational articulation of the same kinds of populism well-utilised by leaders like Margaret Thatcher and Ronald Reagan, both of whom sustained their populist support in two ways: by creating wedges between different marginalised groups and by articulating right-wing programmes based on a false call for individual freedom and individual pleasure together in a way which figured the left as being simultaneously elite, anti-pleasure, anti-individual and as overly focused on an unappealing social conscience and justice framework (Fiske 1989, pp. 163–165). The kind of populism that leads to right-wing dictatorships has also been common for much longer in other parts of the world, including Africa and South America, albeit in somewhat different political and cultural settings.

Populism that takes the form of anti-expertise expresses itself on behalf of the new taxonomy of regimented categories in three specific ways. Firstly, the taxonomy might be said to be a direct backlash not merely to the dominant discourses of sexuality and gender, but to the ways in which they are presented as 'received wisdom' by the figure of the expert and the culture of the institution. There has been a widespread public realisation of what Foucault was first discussing in the 1970s – that medico-legal opinion fabricating itself as expertise and truth (Foucault 2004, p. 42), correlated with institutional controls, mechanisms of supervision and intervention (Foucault 1994, p. 51), has presented categorisations of gender and sexuality in ways which actively produce the figure of the 'abnormal', and that thereby result in injustice and exclusion. This critique of expertise has operated across the entire field of popular cultural politics, from feminism's disavowal of the early popular psychology view of women as automatically irrational and hysterical to the early lesbian/gay activists who sought to argue against the 'expert' idea of non-heterosexuality as an illness that can be cured. Certainly, this populist social justice perspective sponsors the much-needed reversion against decades of medical expertise which unethically and unjustly attempted to make the child who is intersex or the child with 'ambiguous genitalia' *fit* into one or the other of the masculine/feminine gender categories, having seen that which did not fit as an affront to taxonomic classification itself. Yet, there is a kind of populism at play that extends such arguments to question the expertise given by institutions such as sex education, medical and general practice, sexologists and others who articulate the dominant liberal ideas of gender and sexuality, even if those are comparatively benign in contrast to the late nineteenth- and early twentieth-century abnormalisations in gender and sexuality discourse.

Such a populist perspective – somewhat rightly – questions the wisdom of educators, doctors and LGBT rights politicians from a perspective that attempts to supplant expertise that describes how a contemporary man or woman, queer or straight should be, behave and act. This is not, in itself, surprising when the topics of gender and sexuality have been taken up with what Weeks (2017) identified as a "mass democracy" talking endlessly about gender and sexuality "through the globalized media, on television, in chat shows, confessional programmes, soap operas, reality shows, documentaries and advertisements; in cyberspace via social networks, dating and pickup sites and apps, blogs microblogs and vlogs", resulting in a diffusion of expertise (pp. 1–2). One response to this is that we see not only a diffusion of expertise on sex, sexuality and gender, but also a backlash against those who speak in such a way that appears to be an authoritarian or institutional expert speech. The reality television show or the confessional chat show has regularly looked to anomalies in gender and sexuality that operate as 'staged spectacle' in a way which comes to stand in for older realities and in which "sensations is preferable to truth" (Harper 2011, p. 2). While the older realities and truths of gender and sexuality are just as constructed as any new ones, there is a positioning that actively fragments the appeal of the older prompting a search for that which is more spectacular, albeit in ways which, as I have described above, do not go all the way to undoing the authenticity of subjecthood. It is a cautious fragmentation that an anti-expertise sensibility in a populist culture produces around gender and sexuality, doing both the 'good work' of upsetting the norms but at the same time motivated by something which has fundamentally shifted the rational approach to knowledge formation and critique and disavows the nuance and contingency that is sometimes more 'at home' in the discourses of certain elite and expert scholarly knowledge settings.

Secondly, a populist anti-expertise stance disavows the elitism of queer theory, poststructuralism and the fluidity accounts I have described above. This is at least partly because queer theory, which initially distanced itself from expert knowledge within the academy while locating itself academically in such a way as to produce critique (Tierney 1997), is for a newer generation associated with expertise and the liberal elitism of the humanities and social sciences, themselves under attack in many quarters globally. This is not to suggest that all of those who are in favour of the new taxonomy are familiar with queer theory – nor, of course, is it to suggest that queer theory has remained radically contained in the academy, for that is not the case either. Rather, where this older approach to critiquing the discourses of the dominant clashes in concept, in online discussions and in ways of framing futures, it is argued against to some extent as being that which always spoils, much like the feminism Sara Ahmed (2014) described that results in a populist eye-rolling when it says 'no' to that which others take up as natural (p. 154). Like the feminist, queer theory is the killjoy. Indeed, it can be argued that academic queer theory does itself its own disservice through forms of negativity that are at odds with the contemporary cultural discourse of positivism that marks certain North American expressions of identity and agency. Ruti (2017), for example, associates queer theory with a kind of negativity that, while usefully contrasting with the public valorisation of "success, achievement, performance, and self-actualization that characterises today's neoliberal society" (p. 2), simultaneously misses the point that there is a particular love (what Ruti calls "good feelings") that instantly make its argument less appealing among a broader population. In that sense, the anti-fluidity approach of the new taxonomy is more understandable because it has popular appeal and operates in the context of disavowing the nay-saying liberal elitism of academic discourses which undertake a further critique.

The reason for discussing populism is because of the way in which it produces a rhetoric that articulates an opposition to expertise, to liberalism and to the establishment or those who are perceived to have benefitted from the present cultural regime – particularly if they are liberals and experts and urban at the same time. Populism does not emerge as a result of a hatred towards or disappointment in liberal elites; rather, it has always been the product of crisis. As we know from Antonio Gramsci (1971), socio-political organic crises emerge in ways which demonstrate to the public that "uncurable structural contradictions have revealed themselves" (p. 400). The contradiction in this instance is two-fold. Firstly, as I have been arguing, the older regime of gender and sexuality has shown itself to have deep flaws related to inclusion and justice. At the same time, however, LGBT rights and feminism have been associated with a liberal elitism, making the received wisdom of contemporary dominant regimes of liberal gender and sexuality seem suspect. The suspicion is not from the left or from poststructuralist critique as in Marxist feminism or queer theory, but from a clustering of populist arguments that are, in the first instance, opposed to elitism and then secondarily to that which such elites stand for. As Dennis Altman and Jonathan Symons (2016) have pointed out, the landmark articulation in a 2011 speech by Hillary Clinton of the need to extend American-style LGBT rights to fight oppressive regimes around the world suddenly re-makes LGBT people, previously marginalised as the internal enemy, the liberal elite icons of western progressive modernity (p. 132). Simultaneously, of course, such a feminist argument has also been articulated over the past decade, usually in relation to justifying war in Iraq and Afghanistan, again casting some suspicion on versions of liberal feminism that otherwise seemed relatively secure in the west.

Between the critique of the dominant discourses of gender and sexuality (for failing to be inclusive) and the suspicion of these dominant discourses (for their service to a problematic establishment), they are popularly critiqued in the search for something other, a different taxonomy that comes from below. Stuart Hall argued that organic crises, of which this suspicion and criticism are undoubtedly a part, can be *formative*. He described such productive formation in response to crises this way:

> a new balance of forces, the emergence of new elements, . . . new political configurations and 'philosophies', a profound restructuring of . . . ideological discourses . . . pointing to a new result, a new sort of 'settlement' – 'within certain limits'.
>
> *(p. 15)*

Although intended to describe the operations of populist power blocs, this also quite nicely describes the way in which the new taxonomy of gender and sexuality operates as emergent. It has presented a new philosophy of gender and sexuality that is post-binary; it operates in an ideological fashion but also points to the new taxonomy as the 'real' in opposition to false consciousness of the older gender/sexual dichotomies, thereby presenting the new articulation as if a 'truth' (Foucault 1980, p. 118), and it has done so in a way which 'settles with limitations', which is a way of understanding the expanded representation of gender and sexuality labels without the undoing of underlying regimes that demand coherent subjectivity.

Conclusion: an ethics of groundings and release

Much of what I have been discussing in this chapter focuses on subjectivity rather than representation. The argument here is that the taxonomy is not so radical a change because it has not disrupted the cultural demand for coherent, intelligible and recognisable subjects. Indeed, it works more in favour of that cultural need than alternative and marginal discourses that have embraced fluidity. What the new taxonomy does, then, is actively combat the possibility of fluidity, denaturalisation and any other critique that would take away the grounding of intelligibility, fixity and coherence. This is not to say that such a production is inherently malicious or wrong, although as I have argued in Chapter 2, I tend to feel that it is unfortunate because the benefits of poststructuralist critique in forging everyday lives that are built on relationality and belonging rather than subjectivity, categorisation, normativisation and surveillance are potentially more ethical and open greater possibilities for responding to the vulnerable and precarious. Relational approaches are, by nature, anti-categorical because they acknowledge – in a deconstructionist sense – that oppositional or excluded categories of identity are very much part of the category through which one might make an identification (Game and Metcalfe 2011). That which is outside the frame or the border of an identity category is, by the very nature of framing, included within it – not as that which is different but because anything that is different is also a deferral of its incorporation. In that context, the new taxonomy is built on a framework of classificatory strictures that disavows the fluidity of relational, blurred frames. A relational approach, nevertheless, is more ethical because it demands a genuine mutuality that undoes the oppositional setting of the I/You dichotomy (Game and Metcalfe 2011, p. 353). In that sense, it thereby fosters at least the ethical potential of understanding of the other and understanding of otherness itself.

However, in saying this, if we were to disavow the new taxonomy altogether, we would be equally as unethical in the sense that it would be to fail to respond to the very *immediate* needs of those who benefit from the taxonomy the most, such as those whose lives would be unliveable without micro-minoritised categories that better represent felt experiences of gender and sexuality. Ethical responses can happen in more than one temporal framework, and while there is an immediacy at hand – including (I hope) as a grounding that can help prevent suicidality – there is a longer-term ethical response which is to argue that there is a continuing need to address the resource distribution that prevents many from accessing the more beneficial tools of critical theory, poststructuralism, queer theory and other nuanced theoretical and scholarly approaches to making sense of both the conditions and the future possibilities of gender and sexuality. These theoretical approaches are likely unknown to many who have not experienced the privilege of a university education and made particular subject choices to study in the humanities and social sciences (where they remain available), or the resources to make it possible to embrace a scholarly, nuanced, complex set of discourses that can help produce nuanced, responsive, relational and ethical subjectivities beyond the strictures of the demands for the coherent subject.

The new taxonomy is produced in the context of a generation born into digital media use which includes the widespread availability of information, languages, discourses and alternatives; the communicative form of interactive engagement that actively calls for collaboration in the creation of such approaches; the nuances and reflexivities of identities performed in online spaces; and the role of networking to bring together disparate voices of the marginalised. However, as I have been arguing, like all cultural emergences the new taxonomy does not come from nowhere, appearing online as if some alien language planted and appealing. Rather, it is constituted in its responsiveness to perceived cultural needs, and these include the five I have discussed here: the shift from a homophobic discourse to a sexual citizenship which presented the needs, albeit deeply problematic, of neoliberalism in its accompaniment to a rights-based discourse of tolerance; the needs for authenticity that persist despite the many arguments presented in scholarship against it; the needs of those whose genders and sexualities could not be expressed through the more narrow dominant discourses and thereby let too many 'fall through the cracks'; and the arguably populist needs for disavowing fluidity and anti-foundationalist discourses in order to shore up the needs of coherent subjectivity within the contemporary regime. Without trying to apply too much of a value judgement, this discussion is not intended to foreclose on the possibility that the emergent taxonomy of gender and sexuality labels has other uses, some of which may not yet have emerged as significant.

References

Ahmed, S., 2014. *Willful Subjects*. Durham, NC: Duke University Press.

Altman, D., 1971. *Homosexual Oppression and Liberation*. 2nd ed. New York: New York University Press.

Altman, D., 1979. *Coming out in the Seventies*. Sydney, NSW: Wild and Woolley.

Altman, D., and Symons, J., 2016. *Queer Wars*. Cambridge: Polity.

Anderson, B., 1983. *Imagined Communities: Reflections on the Origins and Spread of Nationalism*. 2nd ed. London: Verso.

Anderson, E., 2008. 'Being masculine is not about who you sleep with . . .': heterosexual athletes contesting masculinity and the one-time rule of homosexuality. *Sex Roles*, 58 (1), 104–115.

Bell, L., 2013. Trigger warnings: sex, lies and social justice utopia on Tumblr. *Networking Knowledge: Journal of the MeCCSA Postgraduate Network*, 6 (1), 31–47. Available from: http://ojs.meccsa.org.uk/index.php/netknow/article/view/296/136 [Accessed 18 January 2016].

Belsey, C., 1994. *Desire: Love Stories in Western Culture*. Oxford: Blackwell.

Budick, S., and Iser, W., eds., 1989. *Languages of the Unsayable: The Play of Negativity in Literature and Literary Theory*. New York: Columbia University Press.

Burgess, J., and Green, J., 2009. *YouTube: Online Video and Participatory Culture*. Cambridge: Polity.

Butler, J., 1990. *Gender Trouble: Feminism and the Subversion of Identity*. London: Routledge.

Butler, J., 1991. Imitation and gender insubordination. *In:* D. Fuss, ed. *Inside/out: Lesbian Theories, Gay Theories*. London: Routledge, 13–31.

Butler, J., 1993. *Bodies That Matter: On the Discursive Limits of 'Sex'*. London: Routledge.

Butler, J., 1997. *The Psychic Life of Power: Theories in Subjection*. Stanford, CA: Stanford University Press.

Butler, J., 2005. *Giving an Account of Oneself*. New York: Fordham University Press.

Byron, P., 2015. Troubling expertise: social media and young people's sexual health. *Communication Research and Practice*, 1 (4), 322–344.

Caputo, J.D., 1993. *Against Ethics: Contributions to a Poetics of Obligation with Constant Reference to Deconstruction*. Bloomington, IN: Indiana University Press.

Cohen, A.P., 1985. *The Symbolic Construction of Community*. London: Ellis Horwood and Tavistock Publications.

Cover, R., 2000. First contact: queer theory, sexual identity, and 'mainstream' film. *International Journal of Gender and Sexuality*, 5 (1), 71–89.

Cover, R., 2006. Audience inter/active: interactive media, narrative control & reconceiving audience history. *New Media & Society*, 8 (1), 213–232.

Cover, R., 2010. More than a watcher: 'Buffy' fans, amateur music videos, romantic slash and intermedia. *In:* P. Attinello, J.K. Halfyard and V. Knights, eds. *Music, Sound and Silence in Buffy the Vampire Slayer*. London: Ashgate, 131–148.

Cover, R., 2012a. *Queer Youth Suicide, Culture and Identity: Unliveable Lives?* London: Routledge.

Cover, R., 2012b. Performing and undoing identity online: social networking, identity theories and the incompatibility of online profiles and friendship regimes. *Convergence*, 18 (2), 177–193.

Cover, R., 2014. Becoming and belonging: performativity, subjectivity and the cultural purposes of social networking. *In:* A. Poletti and J. Rak, eds. *Identity Technologies*. Madison, WI: University of Wisconsin Press, 55–69.

Cover, R., 2016. *Digital Identities: Creating and Communicating the Online Self*. London: Elsevier.

Derrida, J., 1978. *Writing and Difference*, trans. A. Bass. Chicago: University of Chicago Press.

Derrida, J., 1985. *Ear of the Other: Otobiography, Transference, Translation*, trans. P. Kamuf. New York: Schocken Books.

Derrida, J., 1989. How to avoid speaking: denials, trans. K. Frieden. *In:* S. Budick and W. Iser, eds. *Languages of the Unsayable: The Play of Negativity in Literature and Literary Theory*. New York: Columbia University Press, 3–70.

Derrida, J., 1996. *Monolingualism of the Other, or the Prosthesis of Origin*, trans. P. Mensah. Stanford, CA: Stanford University Press.

Diamond, L.M., 2008. *Sexual Fluidity: Understanding Women's Love and Desire*. Cambridge, MA: Harvard University Press.

Dobre, C., 2012. *Furries: Enacting Animal Anthropomorphism*. Plymouth: University of Plymouth Press,

Douglas, M., 1966. *Purity and Danger*. London: Routledge.

Dreher, T., 2017. The 'uncanny doubles' of queer politics: sexual citizenship in the era of same-sex marriage victories. *Sexualities*, 20 (1–2), 176–195.

Drucker, D.J., 2012. Marking sexuality from 0–6: the Kinsey Scale in online culture. *Sexuality & Culture*, 16 (3), 241–262.

Duggan, L., 2002. The new homonormativity: the sexual politics of neoliberalism. *In:* R. Castronovo and D. Nelson, eds. *Materializing Democracy: Toward a Revitalized Cultural Politics*. Durham, NC: Duke University Press, 175–194.

Durkheim, E., 1952. *Suicide: A Study in Sociology*, trans. J.A. Spaulding and G. Simpson. London: Routledge and Kegan Paul.

Epstein, S., 1990. Gay politics, ethnic identity: the limits of social constructionism. *In:* E. Stein, ed. *Forms of Desire: Sexual Orientation and the Social Constructionist Controversy*. New York: Garland, 239–293.

Evans, D.T., 1993. *Sexual Citizenship: The Material Construction of Sexualities*. London: Routledge.

Fiske, J., 1989. *Understanding Popular Culture*. London: Unwin Hyman.

Foucault, M., 1980. *Power/Knowledge: Selected Interviews & Other Writings 1972–1977*, ed. C. Gordon and trans. C. Gordon et al. New York: Pantheon.

Foucault, M., 1990. *The History of Sexuality: An Introduction*, trans. R. Hurley. London: Penguin.

Foucault, M., 1994. *Ethics, Subjectivity and Truth*, ed. P. Rabinow and trans. R. Hurley et al. New York: New York Press.

Foucault, M., 2004. *Abnormal: Lectures at the Collège de France 1974–1975*, eds. V. Marchetti and A. Salmoni and trans. G. Burchell. New York: Picador.

Foucault, M., 2007. *Security, Territory, Population: Lectures at the Collège de France, 1977–78*, ed. M. Senellart and trans. G. Burchell. Hampshire: Palgrave Macmillan.

Foucault, M., 2008. *The Birth of Biopolitics: Lectures at the Collège de France, 1978–79*, ed. M. Senellart and trans. G. Burchell. Hampshire: Palgrave Macmillan.

Freud, S., 1979. A child is being beaten. *In: Penguin Freud Library, vol. 10*. London: Penguin, 161–193.

Fuss, D., 1995. *Identification Papers*. London: Routledge.

Game, A., and Metcalfe, A., 2011. Belonging: from identity logic to relational logic. *Continuum: Journal of Media & Cultural Studies*, 25 (3), 347–357.

Gramsci, A., 1971. *Selections from the Prison Notebooks of Antonio Gramsci*, ed. and trans. Q. Hoare and G.N. Smith. London: Lawrence and Wishart.

Griffin, F.H., 2016. *Feeling Normal: Sexuality and Media Criticism in the Digital Age*. Bloomington, IN: Indiana University Press.

Grosz, E., 1989. *Sexual Subversions: Three French Feminists*. Sydney, NSW: Allen and Unwin.

Grosz, E., 1994. *Volatile Bodies: Toward a Corporeal Feminism*. St. Leonards, NSW: Allen and Unwin.

Grosz, E., 1995. *Space, Time and Perversion: The Politics of Bodies*. London: Routledge.

Harper, T., 2011. *Democracy in the Age of New Media: The Politics of the Spectacle*. New York: Peter Lang.

Jameson, F., 1985. Postmodernism and consumer society. *In*: H. Foster, ed. *Postmodern Culture*. London: Pluto Press, 111–125.

Johnson, C., 2017. Sexual citizenship in a comparative perspective: dilemmas and insights. *Sexualities*, 20 (1–2), 159–175.

Kennedy, H., 2006. Beyond anonymity, or future directions for internet identity research. *New Media & Society*, 8 (6), 859–876.

Kral, M.J., 1994. Suicide as social logic. *Suicide & Life-Threatening Behavior*, 24 (3), 245–259.

Leap, W.L., 1996. *Word's out: Gay Men's English*. Minneapolis, MN: University of Minnesota Press.

Lessig, L., 2008. *Remix: Making Art and Commerce Thrive in the Hybrid Economy*. London: Bloomsbury Academic.

Marcuse, H., 1969. *Eros and Civilization: A Philosophical Inquiry into Freud*. New ed. London: Sphere.

McKee, A., 2012. The importance of entertainment for sexuality education. *Sex Education*, 12 (5), 499–509.

Miller, D., and Sinanan, J., 2014. *Webcam*. London: Polity.

Mouffe, C., 1995. Democratic politics and the question of identity. *In*: J. Rajchman, ed. *The Identity in Question*. London: Routledge, 33–45.

Penley, C., 1997. *Nasa/Trek: Popular Science and Sex in America*. London: Verso.

Plummer, K., 1995. *Telling Sexual Stories: Power, Change and Social Worlds*. London and New York: Routledge.

Rasmussen, M.L., 2006. *Becoming Subjects: Sexualities and Secondary Schooling*. London: Routledge.

Ruti, M., 2017. *The Ethics of Option out: Queer Theory's Defiant Subjects*. New York: Columbia University Press.

Savin-Williams, R.C., 2001. A critique of research on sexual-minority youths. *Journal of Adolescence*, 24 (1), 5–13.

Shneidman, E., 1985. *Definition of Suicide*. New York: John Wiley and Sons.

Tierney, W.G., 1997. *Academic Outlaws: Queer Theory and Cultural Studies in the Academy*. Thousand Oaks, CA: Sage.

Weeks, J., 1998. The sexual citizen. *Theory, Culture & Society*, 15 (3–4), 35–52.

Weeks, J., 2017. *Sexuality*. 4th ed. London: Routledge.

Printed in the United States
By Bookmasters